WHAT TO DO WHEN CHILDREN CLAM UP IN PSYCHOTHERAPY

CREATIVE ARTS AND PLAY THERAPY

Cathy A. Malchiodi and David A. Crenshaw
Series Editors

This series highlights action-oriented therapeutic approaches that utilize art, play, music, dance/movement, drama, and related modalities. Emphasizing current best practices and research, experienced practitioners show how creative arts and play therapies can be integrated into overall treatment for individuals of all ages. Books in the series provide richly illustrated guidelines and techniques for addressing trauma, attachment problems, and other psychological difficulties, as well as for supporting resilience and self-regulation.

Creative Arts and Play Therapy for Attachment Problems
Cathy A. Malchiodi and David A. Crenshaw, Editors

Play Therapy: A Comprehensive Guide
to Theory and Practice
David A. Crenshaw and Anne L. Stewart, Editors

Creative Interventions with Traumatized Children,
Second Edition
Cathy A. Malchiodi, Editor

Music Therapy Handbook
Barbara L. Wheeler, Editor

Play Therapy Interventions to Enhance Resilience
David A. Crenshaw, Robert Brooks, and Sam Goldstein, Editors

What to Do When Children Clam Up in Psychotherapy:
Interventions to Facilitate Communication
Cathy A. Malchiodi and David A. Crenshaw, Editors

What to Do When Children Clam Up in Psychotherapy

Interventions to Facilitate Communication

edited by
Cathy A. Malchiodi
David A. Crenshaw

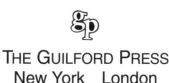

THE GUILFORD PRESS
New York   London

Library of Congress Cataloging-in-Publication Data

Names: Malchiodi, Cathy A., editor. | Crenshaw, David A., editor.
Title: What to do when children clam up in psychotherapy : interventions to
    facilitate communication / edited by Cathy A. Malchiodi, David A. Crenshaw.
Other titles: Creative arts and play therapy.
Description: New York : The Guilford Press, [2017]. | Series: Creative arts
    and play therapy | Includes bibliographical references and index.
Identifiers: LCCN 2017020398| ISBN 9781462530434 (hardcover : alk. paper) |
    ISBN 9781462530427 (paperback : alk. paper)
Subjects: | MESH: Sensory Art Therapies—methods | Child | Adolescent |
    Treatment Refusal | Defense Mechanisms | Communication Barriers |
    Professional–Patient Relations
Classification: LCC RC480.5 | NLM WM 450 | DDC 616.89/14—dc23
LC record available at *https://lccn.loc.gov/2017020398*

About the Editors

Cathy A. Malchiodi, PhD, ATR-BC, LPCC, LPAT, REAT, is an art therapist, expressive arts therapist, and clinical mental health counselor, as well as a recognized authority on art therapy with children, adults, and families. She has given more than 400 presentations on art therapy and has published numerous articles, chapters, and books, including *Understanding Children's Drawings* and *Handbook of Art Therapy, Second Edition.* Dr. Malchiodi is the founder and executive director of the Trauma-Informed Practices and Expressive Arts Therapy Institute. She has worked with a variety of community, national, and international agencies, particularly on the use of art therapy for trauma intervention, disaster relief, mental health, medical illness, and prevention. She is the first person to have received all three of the American Art Therapy Association's highest honors: Distinguished Service Award, Clinician Award, and Honorary Life Member Award. She has also received honors from the Kennedy Center and Very Special Arts in Washington, D.C. A passionate advocate for the role of the arts in health, she is a blogger for *Psychology Today.* Dr. Malchiodi is coeditor (with David A. Crenshaw) of Guilford's Creative Arts and Play Therapy series.

David A. Crenshaw, PhD, ABPP, RPT-S, is Clinical Director of the Children's Home of Poughkeepsie, New York, and Adjunct Faculty at Marist College. He has taught graduate courses in play therapy at Johns Hopkins University and Columbia University and has published widely on child and adolescent therapy, child abuse and trauma, and resilience in children. A Fellow of the American Psychological Association and of its Division of Child and Adolescent Psychology, Dr. Crenshaw is past president of the Hudson Valley Psychological Association, which honored him with its Lifetime Achievement Award, and of the New York Association for Play Therapy. He is currently Chair of the Board of Directors of the Coalition against Sexual and Domestic Abuse and a member of the professional advisory board of the Courthouse Dogs Foundation and of the Dutchess County Task Force against Human Trafficking. He is coeditor (with Cathy A. Malchiodi) of Guilford's Creative Arts and Play Therapy series.

Contributors

Sarah Caprioli, LMHC, private practice, Poughkeepsie, New York

David A. Crenshaw, PhD, ABPP, RPT-S, Clinical Director, Children's Home of Poughkeepsie, New York

Lennis G. Echterling, PhD, Department of Graduate Psychology, James Madison University, Harrisonburg, Virginia

Tracie Faa-Thompson, MA, Turn About Pegasus, Lowick, Northumberland, United Kingdom

Richard L. Gaskill, EdD, Department of Counseling, Educational Leadership, Educational and School Psychology, Wichita State University, Wichita, Kansas

Amber Elizabeth L. Gray, MPH, MA, Restorative Resources Training and Consulting, Santa Fe, New Mexico

Theresa Kestly, PhD, Sand Tray Training Institute of New Mexico, Corrales, New Mexico

Cathy A. Malchiodi, PhD, ATR-BC, LPCC, LPAT, REAT, Trauma-Informed Practices and Expressive Arts Therapy Institute, Louisville, Kentucky

Bruce D. Perry, MD, The ChildTrauma Academy, Houston, Texas, and Feinberg School of Medicine, Northwestern University, Chicago, Illinois

Stephen W. Porges, PhD, Department of Psychiatry, University of North Carolina at Chapel Hill School of Medicine, Chapel Hill, North Carolina

Anne L. Stewart, PhD, Department of Graduate Psychology, James Madison University, Harrisonburg, Virginia

Martha B. Straus, PhD, Department of Clinical Psychology,
Antioch University New England, Keene, New Hampshire

Risë VanFleet, PhD, Family Enhancement and Play Therapy Center,
Boiling Springs, Pennsylvania

Nancy Boyd Webb, DSW, LICSW, RPT-S, Graduate School of Social Service,
Fordham University, Bronx, New York

Preface

Of all the vexing problems that child therapists face, perhaps none creates as much angst in the therapist as a child who shuts down and can't or won't talk. Some child or play therapists would rather deal with a child who trashes the playroom in a rage than a child who won't talk. Why would this be? Perhaps the child who clams up triggers a therapist's fears of inadequacy, incompetence, or impotence because therapy is most often conceived of primarily as a verbal process. Although child therapists typically are soundly grounded in child development, even an experienced child therapist in the process of reflecting and self-monitoring can conclude, "I ask my child clients too many questions." We recognize that verbal communication is not the strong suit of young children, yet in therapy with them, we find ourselves subtly and sometimes not too subtly pressuring children toward a more verbal process. Thus, children clam up. Worse, it has been traditional throughout the history of child therapy to call such "clam-ups" sure signs of resistance to therapy.

This volume, which we are honored to edit, includes highly accomplished therapists' and researchers' explanations of why the concept of resistance doesn't begin to capture the complexity of why children shut down in therapy. The book begins with two introductory chapters by the editors on factors contributing to children's clamming up in therapy and an examination of the concept of resistance in child therapy. Neurobiological contributing factors (Richard L. Gaskill & Bruce D. Perry, Chapter 3; Amber Elizabeth L. Gray & Stephen W. Porges, Chapter 6; and Theresa Kestly, Chapter 7) are explored in depth along with ways of therapeutically addressing these factors in practical terms. Anne L. Stewart and Lennis G. Echterling (Chapter 4) explore the underlying meanings behind children clamming up in therapy and outline a helpful framework for therapists to intervene. In Chapter 5, Nancy Boyd

Webb covers selective mutism as a silencing factor, which can be quite challenging to the child therapist because of the relative rarity of this condition. Martha B. Straus (Chapter 8) writes about the contribution of adolescent attachment trauma. Sarah Caprioli and David A. Crenshaw (Chapter 9) look at cultural factors in silencing children not only in therapy but also in court when children are testifying as witnesses to their own abuse. This volume concludes with an overview of how art therapy can enable therapeutic communication when verbal approaches reach an impasse (Cathy A. Malchiodi, Chapter 10) and an examination of the virtues of Animal Assisted Play Therapy with children when words fail (Risë VanFleet & Tracie Faa-Thompson, Chapter 11).

Unique to this book, with the exception of the overview (Chapter 1), are five recommended practices to guide practitioners in dealing with clamming up from the perspectives of each chapter. This feature provides the reader with clear ideas for the practical, day-to-day world of clinical practice. The editors have found from their prior experience that, although readers appreciate theory and state-of-the-art research, they are most interested in how all of this updated knowledge applies to the clients they are scheduled to see this week. As editors we also encouraged our authors to write their chapters in ways that communicate the practical implications of their considerable and impressive expertise in their designated areas.

In assembling this volume, we were guided by experiences in our early years as child therapists. Because, at that stage, we did not fully understand the complexity of the developmental, temperamental, neurobiological, psychodynamic, family, or cultural factors that make up the complex tapestry of reasons why children may find it hard to verbalize, we plead guilty to resorting to the concept of resistance, which amounted to blaming the child or family for lack of participation or compliance in therapy. Now that we have both engaged children and families for decades, resistance is a dubious concept in our view and in work with clients. We can't help but wish there had been a volume like this one available to us at that time. It would have served our clients well. We hope that it will serve our readers well, and we are grateful to the outstanding contributors to this book for sharing their considerable wisdom and rich experiences in helping children who might otherwise clam up find their voices through verbal expression, play, art, music, drama, dance, or other creative arts.

CATHY A. MALCHIODI
DAVID A. CRENSHAW

Contents

Part I

GENERAL PRINCIPLES
TO GUIDE PRACTICE

Why Children Clam Up in Therapy

Cathy A. Malchiodi
David A. Crenshaw

Children do not always start to verbalize their issues and concerns immediately upon arriving at our offices. While most practitioners understand child development well enough to appreciate this fact, they still may expect children to verbally respond to requests to talk. This often takes the form of asking young clients too many questions instead of allowing them to tell their stories in more child-friendly ways. This response can inadvertently stall the therapeutic process with children who might otherwise share their stories through play-based communication or express their narratives through creativity and imagination.

Clinical experience has taught us children actually long to unburden themselves of disquieting secrets, painful life experiences, hurtful relationships, and traumatic events. They will not talk to us, however, unless the therapeutic context and, more important, the helping relationship is safe, inviting, and comfortable. To this end, the authors in this book describe the variety of reasons why and situations in which children "clam up"—a colloquialism that refers to an individual's silence, often in response to a request to disclose information. According to this definition, one may clam up when nervous, embarrassed, or simply because one does not want to talk about a particular subject, event, or feeling. Crenshaw (2008) notes that children in particular often "hit a wall" for a variety of reasons when asked to talk about their feelings or worries in individual, group, or family therapy. In that moment, the helping professional suddenly is forced to reframe the focus of therapeutic interactions, allow the child to "save face," and discover other ways to help a young client participate in meaningful, productive ways. Most therapists will agree that this is one of the most common challenges in treatment and one that requires specific strategies to not only support a child's sense of safety, but also to establish a relationship that facilitates the child's trust in the recovery process. Another basic necessity is the therapist's way of being with the child or adolescent that conveys the kind of acceptance, warmth, and caring that frees the child to communicate. The therapist also creates a therapeutic space (context) that is engaging, disarming, enveloped in safety, and invites attachment.

Each chapter in this volume provides clinical illustrations of why children may be unable to verbalize during treatment. For example, some are due to strictly developmental issues dependent on a child's age, physical challenges, or cognitive capacities that make words difficult. Other chapters describe children who may struggle with anxiety, fear, or resentment and are unable to verbally articulate emotions or perceptions; for those who have experienced one or more traumatic events, language may be inhibited by a flood of trauma-related memories, avoidance responses, or psychic numbing.

In this chapter, we introduce readers to the central premises of this book and, in particular, why children clam up during treatment. We also establish a foundation to explain how a variety of nonverbal approaches, including play therapy, creative arts therapies, and action-oriented approaches and strategies facilitate effective therapeutic intervention with children who find verbal communication difficult or challenging. Finally, the key characteristics of play therapy and creative arts therapies are explained as essential ways to help children externalize their stories and support verbal narratives.

WHY CHILDREN CLAM UP

There are numerous reasons why children clam up in therapy. Developmental factors such as the child's age, cognitive abilities, and physical challenges may affect if or when a child shares verbal narratives during treatment. For very young children, language is not usually the primary mode for expressing stories or relating life experiences. In addition, temperament can influence the style of a child's communication. Many children, especially during initial therapy sessions, are naturally shy, introverted, or reticent to speak to the therapist until trust and a level of comfort are achieved, efficacy is internalized, and young clients perceive a supportive relationship. While a preference not to speak may be due to many reasons, recent studies indicate that a significant proportion of older children actually describe themselves as "shy," underscoring that disposition and temperament actually span a wide range of "normal" (Burstein, Ameli-Grillon, & Merikangas, 2011).

Culture may also be a factor in children's preferences for verbal communication. Self-expression in therapy may be inhibited by differences in verbal and nonverbal communication in cross-cultural therapy (Sue & Sue, 1977) in addition to the language barrier itself. Also, differences in class-bound values and cultural values may serve as formidable barriers to free and natural communication between children and their therapist (Sue & Sue, 1977). Sue (2015) strongly asserts that "any system of therapy is by its nature ethnocentric or more accurately culture-specific" (p. 361). Therapy is a form of cultural oppression, as Sue (2015) persuasively argues, because it is derived from traditional white Western European psychological thought; whenever we impose a sociocultural-dominant form of therapy on a diverse client population the therapy itself can be a form of silencing. If, for example, we are treating an African American inner-city boy who expresses what Hardy and Laszloffy (2005) describe as a "survival orientation" in his thinking, empirically supported protocols may call for challenging the logic of such thinking, even if the behavior is adaptive to the youth's circumstances and survival. The dominant medical model, with its emphasis on pathology, has led to a narrow focus that often ignores the complexity of human beings, including their strengths and resilience. Such culturally specific forms of therapy, to the extent that they occupy a position of sociopolitical power, can silence other forms of healing, such as non-Western, indigenous practices that emphasize rituals and community participation.

Children are also reluctant to come to treatment and, in many cases, were brought by parents who felt pressured to seek intervention. Most often, however, children seen in treatment are unable or decline to speak for the specific problems that bring them into treatment in the first place—life experiences that are distressing, challenging, and even traumatic. These experiences may leave them emotionally vulnerable, preferring not to talk about the very events that create fears, worries, and sadness. Children who have experienced multiple disruptive events such as neglect, abuse, or insecure attachment may not have experienced positive conditions necessary for not only language development, but also trust in caregivers and helping professionals. In addition, children who have been exposed to interpersonal violence may not want to talk because they must maintain secrecy about abuse or violence in order to feel safe and survive (Malchiodi, 1997, 2014). With these young clients, an offhand comment, a disapproving facial expression, or even a stern tone of voice can trigger a cascade of physiological stress responses that are not under voluntary or conscious control. For example, sexually traumatized adolescents may suddenly break eye contact, look down at the floor, purse their lips, and contort their faces, revealing the bodily agony that such focus precipitates when the discussion centers on past trauma events. It is not because they are unwilling to communicate; instead, physiological defense systems (polyvagal system; see Gray & Porges, Chapter 6, this volume, for more information) have hijacked the ability to communicate and socially engage. In addition, in cases of interpersonal violence, and particularly sexual abuse, a "culture of silence" is established in child survivors (Caprioli & Crenshaw, 2015; see Caprioli & Crenshaw, Chapter 9, this volume, for more information). In brief, this silencing not only originates with family systems and communities, it also is reinforced by criminal justice and court systems that purport to help child victims and, as a result, can challenge even the most skilled therapists.

It also is essential that helping professionals accept children's reticence to talk as a normal response to what are often a series of abnormal experiences they are struggling to repair and master. These responses within the context of therapy are not necessarily statements of dysfunction, but rather expressions of "adaptive coping"; when we view children through a trauma-informed lens (see Malchiodi, Chapter 10, this volume, for more information), we immediately begin to accept their resistance, silence, and avoidance of communication simply as reactions that have helped them to survive. In other words, each child responds to stressful situations, including therapy, with personalized strategies for coping and a preference to remain quiet until ready to speak. Just as there are children who eagerly engage with helping professionals, there are children who do not and whose silence is, in effect, a call for help. They may not speak out of fear, anxiety, or even secrecy; others simply may have given up on talking with adults because they have been hurt or abused by caregivers in the past. For some, years of chronic trauma may have left them psychically numb or with somatic reactions ranging from hyperactivation to dissociation when confronted with questions about "what happened." Others may experience what is often referred to as "speechless terror"—the brain's adaptive mechanism that literally shuts down language when sensory memories of terrifying experiences emerge (van der Kolk, 2014). In all cases, these children demand that we address their reactions through channels other than words alone; in brief, intervention must support alternative pathways for communication, while reinforcing a sense of safety and supportive social engagement that helps these young clients self-regulate and trust the therapeutic alliance.

Contributions during the last two decades of neurobiological research have greatly enhanced our ability to understand and explain what is happening in the brain and body when children are unable to speak. In addition to neurobiology, children's reticence to speak can also be framed through humanistic language and concepts. For example, "social maps" (Garbarino & Crenshaw, 2008) reflect the cumulative experience in the child's social world and highly influences expectations of future experiences. If children grow up securely attached to their primary caregivers, their needs are reasonably met, and they are protected and well cared for, their social maps will include beliefs that the world is a safe place and people are trustworthy and dependable. If, on the contrary, children are not securely attached because caretakers have been unpredictable and unreliable, and they have been exposed to violence and abuse, their social maps will reflect their experience in their social world: beliefs that there is no safety, no one to turn to for protection and support, and a lack of people who can be trusted. A child with this social map would be expected to be guarded and mistrustful in approaching therapy, whereas a child with more secure experiences would more easily see the therapist as trustworthy and the therapy space as safe.

PLAYING AND CREATING: EXPRESSING THE UNSPEAKABLE

Helping professionals often encounter children whose experiences are difficult to express with words; many of these events and memories are terrifying for some. When confronted with horror and brutality, play and creative imagination in childhood can come to a halt; fortunately, this is not always the case, and even under extreme conditions, children often are still able to communicate their stories through action-oriented, sensory-based expression. During the Holocaust, for example, some children played in the shadows of crematoriums or on their way to the gas chambers (Eisen, 1988). In camps like Theresienstadt, young people drew and painted images of tremendous beauty and hope under the guidance of sensitive and supportive adults (Goldman-Rubin, 2000). In all cases, these remarkable individuals used play and creative imagination to cope with the terrifying conditions that surrounded them in the face of imminent death (Eisen, 1988; Volavkova, 1978).

Barring the most inhumane and extreme conditions even in war-torn countries, children consistently seek mastery, relief, and compensation through play and creativity; they express the hurts they experience in startling dimensions and expressions beyond what words can convey. While children may attempt to hide their pain from helping professionals, their hurts ask us to offer them alternative possibilities for communication rather than traditional talk therapy. We also are challenged to meet these children "where they are," respecting the pace of intervention to support safety and trust in the therapeutic relationship. In fact, we often need to not only encourage these children to speak, but also offer options for silent refuge at certain key moments.

In summary, there are many factors that can shut down young people's verbal communication in therapy, including cultural, neurobiological, psychodynamic, and trauma-related effects. When children clam up in the face of these, it is clear that the term "resistance" does not begin to capture the complexity of the contributing influences and contextual features. Both trauma and hyperarousal related to trauma can hijack an individual's ability to communicate. Therapy that is neither culture specific nor sensitive may also inhibit verbal communication in addition to the well-known psychodynamic factors creating conflict and ambivalence about verbal disclosure. When children cannot tell their story in words, even those as young as three can express their inner worlds through play, art, sandtray creations, or other creative arts depictions. The uncanny ability of these children to share their narratives through play, art, music, drama, or with miniature figures in a sandtray underscores both the value of right-hemisphere, implicit communication in therapy and the innate self-reparative capacities of these creative modalities. The following sections provide an overview of these approaches, underscoring how each creatively facilitates communication and expands the possibilities for self-expression within the context of therapy.

PLAY THERAPY

Play therapy is defined as the systematic use of play to help individuals prevent or resolve psychosocial difficulties and achieve optimal growth and development (Webb, 2007; Landreth, 2012) and employs a variety of theoretical orientations, including child-centered, Jungian, Adlerian, and others (Crenshaw & Stewart, 2015). It is nearly as old as the field of psychotherapy itself and is generally used with children, but also with families (Gil, 2015a). More recently, play therapy theory has incorporated emphasis on attachment research and neurobiology (Malchiodi & Crenshaw, 2014). Play therapists use a wide range of creative interventions that include toys, props, games, sandplay, and expressive arts and is very similar in theory and approach to that of arts-based therapists who apply many forms of creative intervention in their work. For example, a play therapist may invite a child to engage in painting or work with clay and then facilitate role play or storytelling through puppets, provide imaginative props, or encourage the use of toy miniatures in a sandbox.

Play is a precursor to creative expression and exploration. Developmentally, play exists before formal artistic expression; in the earliest months of life, infants learn play through rhythm and tempo, social interactions with others through body language and sounds, and experiences like "peek-a-boo" and other sensory-based relationships with caregivers. These experiences, combined with development of cognitive and motor skills, make it possible for children to engage not only in imaginative play, but also in drawing, music making, movement, and pretend activities later on.

Play therapy creates opportunities for children to express untold stories, burdensome secrets, agonizing conflicts, and terror and traumatic events. The setting in which play therapy takes place, the playroom, is an environment that appeals to children, furnished with toys, puppets, sandtrays and miniatures, art supplies, drawing tables, and family playhouses. Play is natural to children and allays anxiety. Therapeutic play allows children to regulate the pace of confrontation with painful material; this is especially true in child-centered play therapy, but all forms of play therapy aim to keep the therapy process safe for the child, and sensitive timing and pacing is the key to that end. Intrinsic qualities of play, such as displacement from action and impulse into symbolic expression, allows the child to gradually approach the most sensitive and painful parts of what hurts internally or within their relational world.

Finally, play is a form of what Schore (2012) describes as right-hemispheric communication that holds the key to emotional regulation. Schore underscores how emotion dysregulation is central to virtually every psychiatric disorder, and action-oriented approaches that include play can help to address this dysregulation in ways that words alone cannot. Play therapy, therefore, occupies a place of great importance in contemporary psychotherapy with children as a result of the interpersonal neurobiological approach elucidated by Perry (2009, 2015), Schore (2003a, 2003b, 2012), and Siegel (1999, 2012).

CREATIVE ARTS THERAPIES

Like play therapy, creative arts therapies can help children bypass the limitations of language as well as expand possibilities for reparative communication through approaches that at least temporarily bypass language (Malchiodi & Crenshaw, 2014). The creative arts (visual art, music, movement, and drama) have an extensively documented and long history of use in self-expression, self-regulation, reparation, and commemoration, with numerous references throughout medicine, anthropology, and the arts to the earliest healing applications of these forms of communication (Malchiodi, 2005, 2015). Specifically, the creative arts therapies are defined as purposeful individual applications of art therapy, music therapy, dance/movement therapy, drama therapy and poetry therapy within a psychotherapeutic framework (Malchiodi, 2007; National Coalition of Creative Arts Therapies Associations [NCCATA], 2016). Expressive arts therapy is defined as the integrative use of creative arts in therapeutic work (Estrella, 2005; McNiff, 2009; Rogers, 2000). The expressive arts therapy approach is generally understood as using more than one art form, consecutively or in combination, although depending on individual or group goals, one art form may dominate a session. In addition, some practitioners use the phrases *integrated arts* or *intermodal therapy* (also known as multimodal) to describe the use of two or more expressive therapies an individual or group session. Because this approach is defined as integrative, intervention is focused on the interrelatedness of the arts with children.

In work with children, several creative arts therapies are often applied individually, within the context of expressive arts therapy or within the use of play therapy. We outline these below.

Art Therapy

Art therapy is the purposeful use of visual art materials and media in intervention, counseling, psychotherapy, and rehabilitation; it is used with individuals of all ages, families, and groups. Within the applications of art therapy, there is a continuum of practice ranging from art as therapy (art making as a reparative, life-enhancing activity; Malchiodi, 2007; McNiff, 2009) to art psychotherapy (the purposeful, integrative application of art-based intervention within a variety of psychotherapeutic and counseling approaches; Malchiodi, 2013). With children, art expression can be both a means of self-regulation as well as symbolic communication of personal stories and worldviews.

Music Therapy

Music therapy uses music to effect positive changes in the psychological, physical, cognitive, or social functioning of individuals with health, behavioral, social, emotional, or educational challenges (Wheeler, 2015). In general, music therapy is applied to work with young clients for affect regulation and communication and to support behavioral and interpersonal goals.

Drama Therapy

Drama therapy is an active, experiential approach to facilitating change through storytelling, projective play, purposeful improvisation, and performance (Johnson, 2009). This active approach helps individuals tell their stories to resolve problems, achieve catharsis, extend the depth of inner experience, and strengthen the ability to understand the self and others. In the context of work with children, applications may include imaginative and play-based uses of toys, props, and puppets to express narratives and communicate symbolic content.

Dance/Movement Therapy

Dance/movement therapy is based on the assumption that the body and mind are interrelated and is defined as the psychotherapeutic use of movement as a process that furthers the emotional, cognitive, and physical integration of the individual and influences changes in feelings, cognition, physical functioning, and behavior (Chaiklin & Wengrower, 2016). With children, dance/movement is used to address a variety of interpersonal, emotional, behavioral, and developmental goals; because it is a dynamic approach, it generally includes the use of music, props, and group processes to achieve therapeutic objectives.

Perry (2015) summarizes the power of both creative arts therapies and play therapy from a modern-day, neurobiology-informed perspective:

> Amid the current pressure for 'evidence-based practice' parameters, we should remind ourselves that the most powerful evidence is that which comes from hundreds of separate cultures across the thousands of generations independently converging on rhythm, touch, storytelling, and reconnection to community . . . as the core ingredients to coping and healing from trauma. (p. xii)

For children, creative expression also serves as a nonverbal means for "breaking the silence" (Malchiodi, 1997) and as a means of "telling without talking" (Malchiodi, 2015) for those who cannot speak publicly about their experiences for various reasons.

PLAY THERAPY AND CREATIVE ARTS THERAPY: POWERFUL PARTNERS IN HELPING CHILDREN COMMUNICATE

There are many reasons play therapy and creative arts therapies are part of the spectrum of recommended practices when addressing children who clam up in therapy. In brief, there are several unique characteristics of these approaches that not only support psychosocial outcomes within therapy, but also stimulate both nonverbal communication as well as language. The following list summarizes the major reasons why these approaches are helpful and effective in work with children who may not be able to communicate their experiences with words alone.

Empowerment

Both play and creative arts therapies are, by their nature, experiences that support empowerment, mastery, and self-efficacy. They stimulate active engagement in the moment and are especially helpful to children who may have been passive victims of toxic circumstances such as abuse, neglect, or interpersonal violence.

Externalization

When children externalize their internal thoughts, feelings, and images, something important happens in terms of mastery. Children reveal compelling facets of their inner world when they play out a drama with puppets, make a picture in a sandtray, draw or paint a picture, create a figure out of clay, or create a play scene in a family playhouse. What gets externalized is experienced as more manageable than what remains internalized. Perry (2015) observes that the fact that the arts, play, and other forms of nonverbal expression are used universally in cultures around the world is significant and underscores their role in health and wellness. There is also evidence that nonverbal expression via action-oriented, sensory-based approaches such as the creative arts may also actually stimulate narrative, thus perhaps reconnecting explicit (story and language) with implicit (sensory) aspects of trauma (Malchiodi, 2013).

Symbol and Metaphor

Both play therapy and art therapy are forms of metaphoric and symbolic communication for children. Because children may seek mastery through play and creative expression when emotions or experiences are overwhelming, these modalities support safe communication through a personal and often idiosyncratic symbolic and metaphoric language. For example, symbolism may be disguised to the degree necessary to allow a child to engage safely in repeated attempts at mastery without getting overwhelmed or disrupted by anxiety. Because children can control play and art making, they remain in control of the timing and pacing of these processes. The child also determines the degree to which the symbolic representation is distant from the actual experience(s). Posttraumatic play (Gil, 2015b) and posttraumatic art expression (Malchiodi, 2014) are also indications of continuing attempts at mastery stemming from the powerful drive to heal and recover from adversity that we call resilience.

Miniaturization

Play therapy and creative arts therapies share in common the offering of opportunities to children to work with their "big problems" that can be experienced as overwhelming in a miniature, more manageable form. For example, working with puppets, putting miniatures in the sand to make a picture, or drawing people or scenes essentially "shrinks" the problem down to a more workable and manageable level for children that enables them to gain mastery.

Playfulness

Play and creative activities are inherently disarming and allay anxiety, enabling children to engage wholeheartedly in mastery, imaginative, and symbolic communication. Play, for example, "takes us out of time's arrow, allows us to exist in a separate 'state' of being from all others . . . but still is a process of being and doing something just for its own sake" (Brown, 2015, p. xi). In brief, play and creative activities can be experiences of joy, possibility, and transformative, yet playful expression.

Containment

Children, as Terr (1983) pointed out, tend to play out or act out their traumatic experiences. We modify the statement, underscoring that children will play, draw, paint, drum, or dance out their most painful experiences including trauma or they will engage in behavioral enactments of these events. There are important advantages to containing the trauma events in symbolic forms of communication rather than a child acting out, for example, sexualized or assaultive behaviors. In other words, containment through play or creative expression can redirect counterproductive behavior enactments that put children at risk for additional emotional pain or punishment

THE IMPORTANCE OF RELATIONSHIP
WITH CHILDREN WHO CLAM UP

While play, creative arts, and other sensory-based or action-oriented approaches can help children communicate their stories when words are too difficult, there is another key factor in the therapeutic equation—relationship. The recent focus on interpersonal neurobiology (Siegel, 2012; see Kestly, Chapter 7, this volume, for more information) underscores its importance as well as explains why relationships heal; similarly, the significance of human interactions via the social engagement system (Porges, 2012; see Gray & Porges, Chapter 6, this volume, for more information) also supports the centrality of how therapists present themselves to their clients with respect to gesture, language and nonverbal, body-based communications. Despite any technique, intervention, or recommended practice, it is the relationship that not only supports children's capacities to self-express, but also is the core factor in all healing.

Relational healing occurs in many ways because each child and helping professional constitute a unique and dynamic relationship. However, it is most often demonstrated to young clients by the therapist's ability to be flexible, playful, and creative in responding to what children bring to treatment. For example, when children respond in their usual way to the therapist, the therapist responds in a different way from what the children have grown to expect. Therapists who are effective in helping children trust the therapeutic process also demonstrate a genuine interest in children's play, imagination, and creative expressions. If the child promises to bring a poem she has written to the next session, the therapist remembers to ask her about the poem early in the next session. If a child shares an important dream in which a particular emotion is symbolized with great intensity, the therapist connects the symbolized affect to an experience shared by the child later in therapy when that same affect was powerfully experienced.

In brief, the therapist who uses play and creative interventions with children is able to convey what Winnicott (1973) reported that "good enough" mothers do or what art therapists have come to call "the third hand," a relational response that recapitulates the positive attachment found in early caregiver–child relationships (Malchiodi, 2015; see Malchiodi, Chapter 10, this volume, for more information). While we can tell children that we are here to support them and help them repair worries and hurts, it is most often our actions (nonverbal cues, sensory-based interactions and gestures) that communicate this support and positive social engagement. In countless past interactions, children who clam up have often come to expect rejection and negative judgments; in contrast, the therapist capitalizing on the "good-enough mother" and "third hand" responds with acceptance and authentic appreciation. The child expects judgment and criticism, the therapist responds with understanding; if an enraged child anticipates a punitive response, the therapist responds with tolerance. In the course of any play- or arts-based psychotherapy with children, the innumerable transactions between child and

therapist ultimately result in an emotionally corrective, relational healing experience rather than any prescribed method, activity, or technique.

CONCLUSION

The premise of this book is based on our belief that nonverbal, action-
oriented approaches are key to helping children who cannot speak
about the unspeakable or decline to talk about their experiences. In
particular, the authors in this volume support the use of play and creative arts as ways to help young clients express what may not be communicated for the various reasons we have summarized in this chapter.
Subsequent chapters in this first section detail the concept of resistance
(Crenshaw) and how neurobiological factors (Gaskill and Perry) affect
young clients' abilities to communicate in therapy. The second section
offers a wide array of wisdom from expert practitioners in the fields
of play therapy, psychology, social work, counseling, and creative arts
therapy, supported by numerous case examples and advanced clinical
experiences. In brief, these experts generously share their knowledge
and diverse approaches to work with a variety of challenges, including
trauma and loss, selective mutism, and disrupted attachment as well as
typical situations in which therapists encounter youth who are reticent
to talk about their feelings or "what happened." Most important, all
chapter authors provide rich and detailed observations, applications,
and recommended practices that demonstrate a variety of practical
strategies that all helping professionals can use to help children and
adolescents who clam up.

REFERENCES

Brown, S. (2015). Foreword. In D. A. Crenshaw & A. L. Stewart (Eds.), *Play
   therapy: A comprehensive guide to theory and practice* (pp. xi–xii). New
   York: Guilford Press.
Burstein, M., Ameli-Grillon, L., & Merikangas, K. (2011). Shyness versus social
   phobia in U.S. youth. *Pediatrics, 128*(5), 917–925.
Caprioli, S., & Crenshaw, D. A. (2015, September 14). The culture of silencing
   child victims of sexual abuse: Implications for child witnesses in court.
   Journal of Humanistic Psychology (online).
Chaiklin, S., & Wengrower, H. (Eds.). (2016). *The art and science of dance/
   movement therapy*. New York: Routledge.
Crenshaw, D. A. (2008). *Therapeutic engagement of children and adolescents:
   Play, symbol, drawing and storytelling strategies*. Lanham, MD: Jason
   Aronson.

Crenshaw, D. A., & Stewart, A. L. (Eds.). (2015). *Play therapy: A comprehensive guide to theory and practice*. New York: Guilford Press.

Eisen, G. (1988). *Children and play in the Holocaust: Games among the shadows*. Amherst: University of Massachusetts Press.

Estrella, K. (2005). Expressive therapy: An integrated arts approach. In C. A. Malchiodi (Ed.), *Expressive therapies* (pp. 183–209). New York: Guilford Press.

Garbarino, J., & Crenshaw, D. A. (2008). Seeking a shelter for the soul: Healing the wounds of spiritually empty children. In D. A. Crenshaw (Ed.), *Child and adolescent psychotherapy: Wounded spirits and healing paths* (pp. 49–62). Lanham, MD: Jason Aronson.

Gil, E. (2015a). *Play in family therapy* (2nd ed.). New York: Guilford Press.

Gil, E. (2015b). Posttraumatic play: A robust path to resilience. In D. A. Crenshaw, R. Brooks, & S. Goldstein (Eds.), *Play therapy interventions to enhance resilience* (pp. 107–125). New York: Guilford Press.

Goldman-Rubin, S. (2000). *Fireflies in the dark: The story of Friedl Dicker-Brandeis and the children of Terezin*. New York: Holiday House.

Hardy, K. V., & Laszloffy, T. (2005). *Teens who hurt: Clinical interventions to break the cycle of adolescent violence*. New York: Guilford Press.

Johnson, D. R. (2009). *Current approaches in drama therapy* (2nd ed.). Springfield, IL: Charles C Thomas.

Landreth, G. (2012). *Play therapy: The art of relationship* (3rd ed.). New York: Routledge.

Malchiodi, C. A. (1997). *Breaking the silence: Art therapy with children from violent homes* (2nd ed.). New York: Taylor & Francis.

Malchiodi, C. A. (Ed.). (2005). *Expressive therapies*. New York: Guilford Press.

Malchiodi, C. A. (2007). *Art therapy sourcebook* (2nd ed.). New York: McGraw-Hill.

Malchiodi, C. A. (2013). Introduction to art therapy in health care settings. In C. A. Malchiodi (Ed.), *Art therapy in health care* (pp. 1–12). New York: Guilford Press.

Malchiodi, C. A. (2014). Art therapy, attachment, and parent–child dyads. In C. A. Malchiodi & D. A. Crenshaw (Eds.), *Creative arts and play therapy for attachment problems* (pp. 52–66). New York: Guilford Press.

Malchiodi, C. A. (2015). Neurobiology, creative interventions and childhood trauma. In C. A. Malchiodi (Ed.), *Creative interventions with traumatized children* (pp. 3–23). New York: Guilford Press.

Malchiodi, C. A., & Crenshaw, D. A. (Eds.). (2015). *Creative arts and play therapy for attachment problems*. New York: Guilford Press.

McNiff, S. (2009). *Integrating the arts in therapy: History, theory, and practice*. Springfield, IL: Charles C Thomas.

National Coalition of Creative Arts Therapies Associations. (2016). About NCCATA. Retrieved July 6, 2016, from *www.nccata.org/#!aboutnccata/czsv*.

Perry, B. D. (2009). Examining child maltreatment through a neurodevelopmental lens: Clinical application of the Neurosequential Model of Therapeutics. *Journal of Loss and Trauma, 14*, 240–255.

Perry, B. D. (2015). Foreword. In C. A. Malchiodi (Ed.), *Creative interventions with traumatized children* (2nd ed., pp. ix–xiii). New York: Guilford Press.

Porges, S. (2011). *The polyvagal theory: Neurophysiological foundations of emotions, attachment, communication, and self-regulation.* New York: Norton.

Rogers, N. (2000). *The creative connection: Expressive arts as healing.* Ross-on-Wye, UK: PCCS Books.

Schore, A. N. (2003a). *Affect regulation and the repair of the self.* New York: Norton.

Schore, A. N. (2003b). *Affect dysregulation and disorders of the self.* New York: Norton.

Schore, A. N. (2012). *The science of the art of psychotherapy.* New York: Norton.

Siegel, D. J. (1999). *The developing mind: Toward a neurobiology of interpersonal experience.* New York: Guilford Press.

Siegel, D. J. (2012). *The developing mind: How relationships and the brain interact to shape who we are* (2nd ed.). New York: Guilford Press.

Stern, D. N. (2010). *Forms of vitality: Exploring dynamic experience in psychology, the arts, psychotherapy, and development.* Oxford, UK: Oxford University Press.

Sue, D. W. (2015). Therapeutic harm and cultural oppression. *The Counseling Psychologist, 43*(3), 359–369.

Sue, D. W., & Sue, D. (1977). Barriers to effective cross-cultural counseling. *Journal of Counseling Psychology, 24*(5), 420–429.

Terr, L. C. (1983). Chowchilla revisited: The effects of psychic trauma four years after a school-bus kidnapping. *American Journal of Psychiatry, 140,* 1543–1550.

van der Kolk, B. (2014). *The body keeps the score: Brain, mind, and body in the healing of trauma.* New York: Viking Press.

Volavkova, H. (1978). *I never saw another butterfly: Children's drawings and poems from Terezín Concentration Camp 1942–1944.* New York: Schocken Books.

Webb, N. B. (2007). *Play therapy with children in crisis* (3rd ed.). New York: Guilford Press.

Wheeler, B. (2015). *Music therapy handbook.* New York: Guilford Press.

Winnicott, D. W. (1973). *The child, the family, and the outside world.* New York: Penguin.

Resistance in Child Psychotherapy

Playing Hide-and-Seek

David A. Crenshaw

Hide-and-seek is a game with great appeal in early childhood in cultures all around the world, and it is played out in many play therapy offices each day. Both the hiding and seeking is invested with emotional significance. The wish to hide oneself or some part of oneself at some point in time is universal. Equally strong is the wish to be found—to know that someone is looking for you and really wants to find you. Young children vary considerably in their ability to endure the suspense about being found, even in the playful context of a hide-and-seek game. Some will call out "I am over here!" because the anxiety about not being found right away is intolerable. D. H. Winnicott (1963/1965) captured the dynamic succinctly when he stated, "Here is a picture of a child establishing a private self that is not communicating, and at the same time wanting to communicate and to be found. It is a sophisticated game of hide-and-seek in which it is a joy to be hidden and a disaster not to be found" (p. 186). Even if the child is in plain sight, a play therapist will often pretend not to be able to find the child in order to build suspense in the playful drama and to challenge the child's ability to delay the gratification of being found. But even when done in small increments some children will get too anxious and suddenly abandon their hiding places.

The anxiety about no one earnestly seeking a missing (hiding) child may be partly rooted in our culture's attitude toward missing children; one government study found that of all runaway/thrownaway children (youth who are asked to leave home by parents), only 21% were reported missing to police or to a missing children's agency for the purpose of locating them (*www.ncjrs.gov/html/ojjdp/nismart/04/ns4.html*). The notion of unreported missing children or children asked to leave by their parents may seem alien to readers in a Western culture that adheres to values of loving and protecting children. But the last statistics available of a national survey (2002) reported 1,682,900 runaway/thrownaway episodes (*www.missingkids.com/en_US/documents/nismart2_runaway.pdf*). The figures for runaway and thrownaway children were combined because a close examination of the statistics suggested that the distinction between runaways and thrownaways was not clear, as many youth had episodes of both kinds.

As children get older, the logistical difficulty of making themselves invisible in the relatively small space of the playroom frequently leads to a modification of the game so that a puppet or other small object is hidden and becomes the focus of the seeking. A playful game of hide-and-seek with a puppet led to a breakthrough in a case of selective mutism I treated, with the elements of playfulness, surprise, and humor playing a role in enabling the child to speak aloud for the first time in therapy (Crenshaw, 2007). The child was hiding a dog puppet from me, but in a playful surprise, upon finding the puppet, with great excitement, I shouted, "I found your monkey!" Immediately, the child exclaimed loudly, "That's not a monkey, that's a dog!" It was the first time the child had spoken in the session and led to her talking regularly in the sessions and gradually at school with her teacher and classmates.

A SUBTLE VERSION OF HIDE-AND-SEEK

Before children will talk about personally difficult things, including matters that cause shame, embarrassment, pain, and humiliation, they need to believe that the adult really wants to hear what they are being asked to disclose. This is true with respect to a therapist in an individual session and to a parent in a family session (Fussner & Crenshaw, 2008). In other words, the parent in a family session or a therapist in an individual session must convince the child they really want to hear (to seek) what the child wants to tell. Implicit in the convincing process is that the parent or therapist not only wants to hear but also is ready to hear whatever the disclosure may be. Otherwise, children will not talk (hide). The child is "hiding," but in this instance the "seeker" is not sufficiently earnest and determined to make it safe for the child to disclose. The lack of safety may be the result of the child fearing that she/he will not be believed or, even worse, blamed, or that the family member or therapist will not be able to handle the disclosure.

Recent surveys (see Lyon, 2014, for a review) reveal that among adults who acknowledge being sexually abused as children, only 10% disclosed during childhood. It is unknown what proportion of the 90% that did not disclose were in therapy at some point during their childhood, but it can be assumed that a number of these victims were hiding while the therapist did not seek in a convincing way. Two of the surveys asked respondents what inhibited disclosure (Anderson, Martin, Mullen, Romans, & Herbison, 1993; Fleming, 1997); the most common reasons included embarrassment, shame, and expectations that they would be blamed or not believed. As is typical of children, respondents also mentioned wanting to protect or fearing punishment from the perpetrator (Caprioli & Crenshaw, 2015). They also mentioned wanting to avoid upsetting others, and not wanting to focus on the abuse themselves. All of these motives can play a role in "hide-and-seek" in child therapy.

RESISTANCE TO THE CONCEPT OF RESISTANCE IN CHILD PSYCHOTHERAPY

Children are often less than enthusiastic about being taken to see a therapist. Gil and Crenshaw (2015) stated:

> Sometimes children have the sense that they are being forced into therapy and don't have much of a choice in whether they participate. As mentioned above, children do not usually seek therapy themselves, with some notable exceptions of older children or teens who are able to verbalize their distress and ask for therapy. Usually, children have varied degrees of hesitancy; the expression of children's disagreement can range from behaving towards therapists in mildly annoying to downright rude ways! (p. 68)

Older children and adolescents often engage in face saving behaviors and protest going to therapy but when the door is closed to the therapy room, they may engage in a wholehearted way. Gil and Crenshaw (2015) explained:

> In our experience, sometimes children and youth put up a front, a kind of dramatic play, expressly designed to show their dissatisfaction with their parents and to assert who is really in control. We have had the experience of children coming in with slouched postures, smelly, belching or farting, avoiding eye contact, and/or looking disinterested (hiding), only to

be surprised by how quickly things change in the therapy office. Clinical understanding, patience, and empathy (seeking) play a big role in helping children's hesitancy decrease. For example, sometimes a simple, "I know how you feel, I hate to do things just because someone else tells me to do them," or "I hate doing things when I'm forced to do them," could change the atmosphere in the room. It's also useful to tell kids that you're "sorry" that this feels so difficult and reassure them that you'll do your best to make the time go by more quickly . . . you are, after all, there to help them, even if that means helping them deal with not wanting to be there! (p. 68)

Resistance (hiding) is frequently regarded as an unwelcome factor in the psychotherapy process. The concept of resistance brings to mind many questions. Resistance to what? Resistance to whom? Is the resistance to the psychotherapy as a whole? Is the resistance only to exploring certain sensitive issues in the therapy? Is the resistance located in the child? Is the resistance located in the therapist? Is the resistance located in both therapist and child? When resistance becomes evident, is it a good thing or a bad thing? Does resistance result from the therapist's agenda differing from the child's or family's agenda? Is resistance a valid concept at all? These are questions to struggle and agonize over, but too important to dismiss even if the answers are elusive.

My much-admired colleague Eliana Gil (Gil & Crenshaw, 2015) also expressed reservations about the concept of resistance. She wrote:

In addition, I have found that using the term *resistance* suggests an adversarial relationship in which the clients are pushing against clinicians directly, in negative (combative) fashion. In fact, resistance is a necessary and appropriate defense that often makes sense in light of what we are inviting children to do: We are asking them to share their deepest thoughts and feelings with strangers, to plunge into deep, dark secrets immediately, in order to then invite them to undertake a course of therapy that we believe might be helpful to them, but usually painful nevertheless. In fact, many of our child clients can't trust these types of invitations with reassurances of safety. It is the clinician's job to become trustworthy to the clients, and once that is achieved, children may feel comfortable beginning to peel the onion, revealing more and more of their true selves. Thus about 10 years ago, I discarded the word *resistance* and now use alternative words such as *ambivalence, uncertainty, hesitancy,* or *reluctance.* When I use these words, I feel differently about my clients and what's going on in the therapy process, and convey a different, more accepting therapeutic posture. (pp. 25–26)

Another esteemed colleague and internationally acclaimed art therapist, Cathy Malchiodi, also is skeptical about the concept of resistance. She stated in her wonderful book *Children's Drawings:*

I rarely find that children are resistant to drawing. I think that extensive experience in both art therapy and clinical counseling helps me to make the art process interesting and appealing to children. One intuitively knows what is exciting and appealing to children. One intuitively knows what is exciting about art making and children will get caught up in the therapist's enthusiasm. (1998, p. 57)

Conversely, Malchiodi points out that if the therapist is uncomfortable and inhibited with art, never enjoyed drawing or painting, or lacks ability or interest in creative expression, this lack of enthusiasm will invariably be communicated to the child (failure to seek), and the child may be reluctant to engage in art expression (hide). Children often take their cues from the therapist.

One of the reasons that I am resistant to the concept of resistance in child psychotherapy is discovering during my evolution as a child therapist that what I initially saw as resistance in children and adolescents (from this point on in the chapter, the term *children* will refer to both children and adolescents), I no longer do. I now view those impasses or setbacks in therapy not as an unwillingness to communicate or participate in the therapy process, but simply my own lack of skills and tools at that point in my development that would have enabled them to communicate with me and participate in the therapy process. I no longer view those children as clamming up because they didn't *want to* communicate but rather that they simply *couldn't* communicate. I didn't know how to structure the therapeutic context in such a way that enabled them to communicate, so they clammed up.

As the years have passed and I've acquired more experience and skill, I rarely encounter what I would consider a resistant child. Of course, there are exceptions to every generalization.

A NOTABLE EXCEPTION: MANDATED CLIENTS

Some children who are mandated by courts to attend therapy may be furious at the very idea of meeting with a therapist and may refuse to cooperate from the outset. Even in these extreme circumstances, I have learned a valuable way ("surviving the rage") of working with such youth from a colleague (Heather Butt, LMSW) at the Children's Home of Poughkeepsie. "Surviving the rage" is a concept that builds on the pioneering work of Winnicott (1951) on hate and rage in the therapeutic process, including the therapeutic relationship. In "surviving the rage," the therapist assumes that the rage has a rational basis rooted in the child's life experiences. The therapist further assumes that there is no more appropriate place than the therapy space to explore and express the rage. Sufficient mutual trust must be developed to allow the youth to feel the therapist can tolerate and contain the rage, and the therapist can trust that both youth and therapist can be kept safe during the journey. It is not expected that the process will be pretty or that in the course of expressing the profound rage, the youth will always use the King's English in verbalizing the raw emotions that may have been smoldering for years. The primary objective is simply surviving the rage and still being there when the rage, now validated and honored, begins to diminish. By "surviving" (the therapist serving as a safe container for the rage), the youth learns that this hostility, perhaps fully justified or at least understandable, need not destroy the self or the other. The therapeutic value is rooted in this accomplishment, which under these circumstances is a major breakthrough. This is no easy feat. It takes courage on the part of both the youth and the therapist and a huge leap of faith and trust in each other.

Stanley Brodsky (2011) wrote an interesting and creative book on reluctant or mandated clients, although it focuses on adults. Brodsky explains how the typical skill set of the therapist—consisting of reflecting, probing, and supporting—often falls short with individuals who do not voluntarily enter therapy or once there do not engage with the therapist. Brodsky particularly argues that the inquiring approach to therapy, with its frequent questioning of the client, can be experienced as intrusive for poorly motivated clients. Brodsky suggests that therapists refrain from questioning the client and instead make assertive statements about what is happening in the client's life, identify behaviors, and describe choices the client might make.

Motivational interviewing (Miller & Rollnick, 1991), while originally studied primarily in adult work, particularly with addictive behavior, is another approach increasingly used with reluctant or poorly motivated adolescents in treatment (Nagy, 2010). Nagy explained that dealing with resistant and risk-taking youth can be taxing for the child and adolescent mental health specialist. When the young patient is engaged in behaviors, such as substance abuse, sexual risk-taking, or driving fast cars, that are positively reinforced by social, developmental, or biological conditions, Nagy suggested that it may be particularly difficult to motivate change. Motivational interviewing (seeking) can raise problem awareness and facilitate change exploration with individuals who may be resistant (hiding), stuck, or not yet open to making behavioral changes. Motivational interviewing draws on a client-centered, collaborative approach, but entails a particular set of principles and skills and techniques described by Miller and Rollnick (1991).

Increasingly, a mindfulness (seeking) approach to working with children and adolescents has been proposed to reduce resistance (hiding) in high-risk adolescents (Himelstein, 2013). Resistance is reframed as "patterns of protection," with the intent to transform forces of opposition into meaningful engagement. Himelstein views mindfulness as a standalone approach, or it can be used in conjunction with other approaches to therapy.

COULD RESISTANCE BE AN IATROGENIC EFFECT OF CHILD PSYCHOTHERAPY?

Child therapists tend to be well-intended, good-hearted, compassionate, and dedicated people, but that doesn't preclude mistakes. When the therapy causes unintended effects, what is sometimes referred to as iatrogenic outcomes, the therapy itself may produce the resistance (hiding). Some child clients may be so strongly opposed to the concept of psychotherapy from the outset that, no matter how well handled the therapy or how skilled the therapist, nothing helpful or productive will occur. But it is important to examine the conduct of the therapy and the strength of the therapeutic alliance, since these are variables that therapists can influence even as other factors may be outside of their control. More than seven decades of psychotherapy outcome research has affirmed the key role of the quality of the therapeutic relationship. The first place to look when "resistance" is encountered is the strength or lack thereof in the therapeutic alliance. Some common pitfalls to be examined are delineated below.

Failures of Therapeutic Presence

Although Carl Rogers along with other humanistic psychologists like Rollo May and Clark Moustakis emphasized our "way of being" with clients, therapeutic presence has not received the focus it deserves in contemporary psychotherapy writings because of the emphasis on the technology (techniques, strategies, interventions) of therapy. Recent papers (Crenshaw & Kenny-Noziska, 2014; Gellar & Porges, 2014) have highlighted the importance of presence—being with clients in a fully attuned, unguarded, receptive, and nonjudgmental way—from both a psychotherapeutic and neurobiological framework.

Failures of Timing and Pacing

Another often-undervalued skill in the conduct of therapy, especially in today's world of briefer forms of therapy, is timing and pacing, a skill that can't be developed in the abstract but only from extensive experience and competent supervision. Improper timing and pacing (while seeking) can result in negative therapeutic reactions that may be incorrectly labeled resistance (hiding). Timing and pacing are especially crucial in trauma-informed therapy. In order for therapy to be productive and healing, the child needs to feel safe physically, psychologically, and even viscerally (van der Kolk, 2014). Safety to a large measure depends on sensitive, empathic timing and pacing. Bessel van der Kolk (2014) makes this point eloquently:

> Confusion and mutism are routine in therapy offices: We fully expect that our patients will become overwhelmed if we keep pressing them for the details of their story. For that reason we've learned to "pendulate" our approach to trauma, to use a term coined by my friend Peter Levine. We don't avoid confronting the details, but we teach our patients how to safely dip one toe in the water and then take it out again, thus approaching the truth gradually. (2014, p. 245)

While this observation was made with respect to adult therapy, I would maintain that sensitive timing and pacing, thereby making the therapy safe, is even more crucial with children.

Anita, a 17-year-old with an extensive sexual trauma background that included familial abuse and, in her early teens, commercial sexual exploitation, was remarkably sweet, personable, responsive, and cooperative. When approaching (seeking) the overwhelmingly painful details of her abuse, however, she would suddenly break eye contact, stare at the floor, and start pursing her lips. She moved into a different psychological space where she was unreachable, unable to verbalize, frozen in time (hiding). Sometimes it was possible for her to write about what she was feeling at those times, and other times not. At times she was able to access "islands of safety" within her body (van der Kolk, 2014, p. 245) that enabled her to continue with the work of integrating her trauma, and sometimes not. At times she was able to develop her trauma narrative utilizing expressive arts techniques such as the Heartfelt Coloring Card strategies (Crenshaw, 2007) by identifying the people who had hurt her and writing notes in the cards to each of them as well as to the one person whom she trusted and who helped her during her nightmarish journey. Throughout the course of the trauma-informed therapy with Anita, timing and pacing (seeking) was a matter of great delicacy and sensitivity in order to keep the therapy safe for a youngster whose sense of trust and safety had been demolished by the "wrecking ball" of her traumatic sexual experiences. If at any point she had broken off therapy while approaching the traumatic experiences, I would not have viewed it as resistance but rather as failures of timing and pacing, and failure to maintain safety in the therapy.

Lack of Clarity about Purpose and Goals

Sometimes what we see as resistance is the result of the therapist having a different agenda than the child client or the family. One compelling feature of the shorter-term therapies that currently predominate—including some that are evidence based, such as the cognitive-behavioral approaches—is the clarity of purpose and goals. Consumers of psychotherapy, including the families of our child clients, are seeking clear goals, objectives, and methods. Families and the children as well often want to know how long therapy will last and what it is intended to accomplish. If there is a failure to communicate on the part of the therapist or confusion or disagreement about what the goals and/or methods (seeking) should be, this could precipitate what might be wrongly viewed as resistance (hiding).

Failure of "Deep Hearing"

It is ironic that the push by third-party payers for briefer forms of therapy can limit hearing and listening in depth to our patients, long a basic cornerstone of therapy. It is astonishing that, given the essential nature of empathic, sensitive, and attuned listening to psychotherapy and the therapeutic relationship, that a journal article, "In Defense of Listening" (Graybar & Leonard, 2005), would need to be written. The authors explain:

> We believe at its most basic level listening is a function of time and intention. Having the time to listen, but not the intention is one problem. Having the intention, but not the time is yet another. We suspect, in fact it is our thesis, that both time and intention to listen are frequently lacking in brief, manualized, and/or biological treatments. A clinician may have the intent to listen, but without time intention is of little worth. Worse, we fear some brief treatments have begun to diminish practitioners' intent to listen. The very nature of many brief manualized and/or medical interventions does not allow for extended periods of empathic listening, listening that allows clients to reveal rather than state their concerns. Instead, clients are forced by the pace and focus of such treatments, often in their first session, to describe themselves and their problems as if they knew and understood both in their entirety. Such expectations set an incredibly low ceiling for listening. It limits our understanding of clients as well as our appreciation for them. (p. 5)

Carl Rogers (1995) elaborated on his concept of "deep hearing":

When I can really hear someone, it enriches my life. Hearing "deeply" means to hear the words, the thoughts, the feeling tones, the personal meaning, even the meaning that is below the conscious intent of the speaker. (p. 8)

If our child clients do not feel we are really listening—perhaps hearing the words but not the meaning of what they are saying—they are likely to respond poorly in some cases by refusing to share with us their deeper feelings and concerns (hiding). If we were to consider such reactions to be resistance, we would be missing the essential point.

Failures of Empathy

Empathic failure can take many forms. For example, the therapist may grasp intellectually the nature of the child's problem and communicate this understanding to the client but in a sterile, cerebral manner that leaves the child feeling that the therapist doesn't really appreciate her/ his experience. It is also possible that the therapist focuses so intently on the feelings of the child that she/he loses objectivity and perspective, which may compromise the therapist's ability to help the child. The therapist may be accurate in the cognitive appraisal of the child's situation and empathize with the feelings (seeking), but may not be viscerally or bodily moved by the child's experience. In this instance, one particularly astute adolescent referred to the therapist as "overtrained." If any of these forms of empathy failure occur, the child may be reluctant to further engage in the therapy or risk disclosure of sensitive issues (hiding). It would be a mistake to label such a reaction as resistance.

Misinterpreting Resistance in Other Forms

When women with histories of childhood sexual traumas and neglect are in treatment, Nussbaum (2010) observed that terrors, including posttraumatic stress reactions, may be aroused. Nussbaum explained that, as children and adolescents, they were forced to submit to the needs of others in order to obtain some token of love and shelter. In adult life, these women may act submissively, relinquishing more assertive, autonomous, and authentic strivings. Nussbaum cautioned that it is imperative that we do not automatically define a seemingly defiant stance as resistance, when actually it may be the healthy manifestation of a striving for independence and assertiveness that indicates developmental advancement.

When healthy strivings of any kind are misconstrued as resistance, we will do our child clients a disservice.

Some conditions that are difficult to treat may be blamed on the client in the form of "resistance." Segal (2010) argues that maladaptive behavior that repeats, typically known as repetition compulsion, is one of those intransigent conditions. Segal explained that repetition compulsion typically does not achieve mastery, rarely resolves without therapeutic intervention, and can be challenging to overcome in psychotherapy. He proposed a new framework, whereby such behavior is divided into behavior of nontraumatic origin and traumatic origin, with some overlap between the two sources. Segal explained that repetitive maladaptive behavior of nontraumatic origin arises from an evolutionary-based process whereby patterns of behavior frequently displayed by caregivers and compatible with a child's temperament are acquired and repeated. Such behavior has a familiarity and egosyntonic aspect that strongly motivates the person to retain the behavior. By contrast, repetitive maladaptive behavior of traumatic origin is characterized by defensive dissociation of the cognitive and emotional components of trauma, making it very difficult for the person to integrate the experience. Repetitive maladaptive behavior's strong resistance to change should not be misinterpreted as the client opposing change or resisting therapy. Such misinterpretations would be rife with countertransference implications and introduce complicating factors into the therapeutic relationship.

Failure to appreciate the dynamic factors that can slow the process of change may also be mistakenly viewed as clients' uncooperative, oppositional attitudes or resistance to psychotherapy. The late Walter Bonime, from whom I received private psychoanalytic supervision for more than a decade, delineated the anxiety that accompanies change and the threat to the sense of self that the change process entails. Bonime (1989) elucidated how change can be threatening because our sense of self is derived from a familiar sense of sensate, cognate, and affective functioning. Any change in that familiar way of functioning, even when the change is positive, can be subjectively experienced as "not me." The result of that shift from the familiar way of functioning is anxiety. Bonime frequently stated in supervision that we are all familiar with the idea of "home sweet home." He stated that home is our pathology, and when we leave that familiar place, no matter how much misery it may cause, to enter unfamiliar territory, we become anxious because it is "not me."

Family therapists have long appreciated the consequences of change; Peggy Papp's (1983) *The Process of Change* is a classic on the subject. She wrote about the complicated process of change:

The central therapeutic issue is not how to eliminate the symptom but what will happen if it is eliminated; the therapeutic argument is shifted from the problem, who has it, what caused it, and how to get rid of it, to how the family will function without it, what price will have to be paid for its removal, who will pay it, and whether it is worth it. (p. 13)

The late Olga Silverstein, Peggy Papp's colleague at the Ackerman Institute for the Family in New York City for many years, was a master of working with families around the consequences of change. I attended many workshops given by Silverstein because I greatly admired her incomparable wisdom and her finely honed skills as a family therapist. I dedicated a book to Olga Silverstein (Crenshaw, 2008), and before her death we had a final, cherished conversation when she and Peggy Papp were honored for their contributions to family therapy by Hunter College in 2009. On numerous occasions I observed Olga work with a family to whom she would make explicit both the positive and negative consequences of change. Like Dr. Bonime, Olga appreciated the threat and anxiety that a change, even a positive one, in family functioning could cause. When exploring the positive consequences of change with a family, there would be no hesitation, and various family members would recite to Olga the benefits of the change. When she would inquire about the negative consequences of change, however, often there would be silence. Olga would always insist that there would be a downside to the change and push the family to identify and state what some of the negative effects might be. If, for example, the school-avoidant son in the family is staying home to keep an eye on his depressed mother and suddenly goes back to school, who is going to take care of the mother? What shifts in the family might that cause? By bringing these opposing, silent forces out into the open, the family then could make an informed decision about the change they were seeking. Also, the family was less likely to be tripped up by their own reluctance to change by making it conscious to all. Olga would also sometimes caution the family to go slow with the changes they were seeking so as to not create too much disruption in the usual way the family functioned. Failure to appreciate the dynamics of the change process may result in therapist frustration and negative feelings in the countertransference that could damage the outcome of therapy.

WHEN WORDS ARE UNABLE TO TELL THE STORY

Preschool children are not expected to come into our offices sit down in a chair and start verbalizing their concerns and issues. While most clinicians understand child development well enough to appreciate this fact, it sometimes happens that, even when doing play therapy or art therapy or some form of expressive arts, therapists will fall back to their comfort zone (depending on their training) and demand of the child a more verbal process. This often takes the form of asking children too many questions instead of allowing them to tell their story in the more developmentally suitable and natural way, through play or the creative arts. This can inadvertently shut down children who might otherwise play out their narratives or express their stories through the creative arts. The interest in play therapy in the United States has grown enormously in the past three decades, with the Association for Play Therapy counting more than 6,000 members and the number of Registered Play Therapists and Registered Play Therapist-Supervisors (highest level of training and experience) grows each year. Some of the unique facets of play therapy that enable young children to create their narrative in a natural way through play include the following.

Symbolic Play

Children seek mastery through play when experiences or emotions are overwhelming. The symbolism may be disguised to the degree necessary to allow a child to safely engage in repeated attempts at mastery without getting overwhelmed or disrupted by anxiety in the play.

Posttraumatic Play

Each self-initiated exposure to a symbolic representation of the traumatic loss or event allows graded and safe exposure in keeping with the exposure component of trauma-focused cognitive-behavioral therapy (TF-CBT) protocols. Since children can break off the play at any moment they remain in control of the process (the timing, and the pacing). The child also determines the degree to which the symbolic representation is distant from the actual experience(s). Posttraumatic play is also an indication of continuing attempts at mastery stemming from the powerful drive to heal and recover from adversity that we call resilience.

Metaphor

Metaphor is a symbolized form of condensed but precise communication. Play and art therapists are taught to "stay within" the metaphors created, rather than make jarring verbal interpretations of similarities between the metaphors and real life.

Externalization

When children externalize thoughts, feelings, and images that reside internally, something important happens in terms of mastery. Children externalize compelling facets of their inner world when they play out a drama with puppets, make a picture in a sandtray, draw or paint a picture, create a figure out of clay, or create a play scene in a family play-house. What gets externalized is experienced as more manageable than what remains internalized.

Miniaturization

Play therapy and expressive arts therapies all offer opportunities for children to work with their overwhelming "big problems" in a more manageable, miniature form. The act of working with puppets, putting miniatures in the sand to make a picture, or drawing people or scenes "shrinks" the problem down to a more workable size for children that enables them to gain mastery.

Playfulness

Play is inherently disarming and allays anxiety, enabling children to engage wholeheartedly in mastery, imaginative, and symbolic play. Highly anxious children or severely traumatized children don't play.

PLAYING THROUGH THE UNSPEAKABLE

Some experiences are too terrifying to be expressed in words. Under conditions of extreme horror and brutality play may even stop, but not always even under such extreme conditions. During the Holocaust, some children played in the shadows of the crematoriums or on the way into the gas chambers (Eisen, 1988). But they were the exceptions. These remarkable, courageous children played "gas chambers" and "funeral carts" in an attempt to cope with the terrifying conditions and their knowledge of imminent and certain death (Eisen, 1988; Volavkova, 1978).

Conditions were so harsh in the ghettos and concentration camps that most malnourished children ill with typhoid—their bodies bro-ken down—no longer played. Barring the most inhumane and extreme conditions, however, even in war-torn countries, children seek mastery, relief, and compensation through play. Sometimes children hurt in places where the pain is of such startling dimensions that words can't reach. When inexpressible pain is at the heart of the child clamming up, more vigorous *seeking* is called for from the therapist, although with respect for the pace that keeps the therapy safe for the child and sensitive timing to the child's need to *hide* at certain key moments.

Verbal expressive language sometimes can't begin to tell the story. Three children, ages 6, 5, and 3 enter the playroom. The oldest child was willing to sit in a circle on a rug with my interns and me. The two younger ones, although they knew the routine, wanted no part of it. They went from activity area to activity area in the playroom, making as much racket and disruption as possible; repeated efforts to get them to join us in the circle for a self-calming exercise that they so desperately needed was met with dramatic escalation. Then the situation became chaotic, bordering on dangerous, as the 3-year-old went around the circle trying to kick each one of us; at the same time, the 5-year-old was turning over the puppet theater and the chairs in the room. Looking around at the wrecked room, furniture turned over, and the oldest child crying because he had been accidently hit in the corner of his eye by his brother's careless and reckless actions, it immediately occurred to me that what the younger two children had just done was to give us front-row seats to a dramatic enactment of their lives. The children had been exposed to chaotic conditions in the home and they had witnessed chronic domestic violence. Part of the chaos of their prior lives consisted of being on the run with their mother, who was trying to escape the child protection authorities looking to remove the children due to lack of safety and structure in the home. What the children demonstrated for us so clearly was the only family life they had known, punctuated by violence, unpredictability, extreme anger, and overriding anxiety and fear. The children were not able to tell their story in words, but they did so in behavioral enactment and play action with a precision that no words could match.

TRAUMA NARRATIVES TOLD THROUGH SYMBOLIC PLAY

The oldest of the three children in the example above, Raul, did something in the playroom on a more symbolic level than the play action engaged in by his siblings. In a subsequent individual play session, once in the playroom he wanted to play doctor with me as his first patient. As doctor, this 6-year-old said that he could help me but he would have to kill me first. He explained that he had to take all the "bad blood" out in order to put the "good blood" in. He took this theme a step further, when I asked the doctor if he could also help my animals. I brought my dog to Dr. Raul first, and then the pet monkey. In all three cases, Dr. Raul said he had to do the same thing (kill them first before he could help them by taking the "bad blood" out then putting the "good blood" in). But he also said that exchanging the blood would not be enough. He would also have to remove their "bad heart" in order to put a "good heart" in.

This young child was not able to tell me how tainted and stigmatized he felt that both of his parents were in prison and that he was convinced that he was a "bad seed" exemplified by "bad blood" and a "bad heart." But he was able to articulate this insidious belief of a condemned self within his play that spoke volumes. His play also expressed a hopeful element. Although the solution was extreme, there was something that could be done about the "bad blood" and the "bad heart." Although play therapists get no training in performing heart transplants or blood transfusions, we do know how to provide experiences in the context of a therapeutic relationship that highlight the virtue and goodness of children that, over time, can modify such damaging beliefs about self as Raul held.

An 11-year-old girl who had suffered sexual trauma of which she was unable to speak lined up in the sandtray all the domestic animals—dogs, cats, cows, horses, goats, and pigs—and pointed them in the same direction. When asked if she wanted to say anything about her picture in the sand, she simply stated, "They are leaving town to go to a different town where they hope they will be treated better!" Words pale in their ability to tell the trauma story compared to the picture this child made in the sand.

THERAPEUTIC PRESENCE, RELATIONAL HEALING, AND RESISTANCE

Children are unlikely to resist (hide) when the therapeutic context is safe and the therapist conveys sincere respect and heartfelt concern for the child, and relates to the child in a fully present, receptive, unguarded, and nonjudgmental manner, which can be viewed as therapeutic presence (Crenshaw & Kenney-Noziska, 2014). In work with children, a complicating factor can be the notion that "as adults we always know best," which not only can alienate the child, but also we may stop listening. When a child feels safe in the presence of a warm, empathic, and genuine therapist, is there any reason to resist (to hide)? Therapeutic presence also takes the form of appreciating the child's reluctance or ambivalence and fully accepting it as a natural protective, adaptive response, thereby rendering such protective measures unnecessary.

When children respond in their usual way to the therapist and the therapist responds differently from what the children have grown to expect, relational healing can happen. If the child promises to bring a poem that she has written to the next session, the therapist remembers (to the child's surprise) to ask her about the poem early in the next session. If a child shares an important dream in which a particular emotion is symbolized with great intensity, the therapist remembers to connect the symbolized affect to an experience the child shares later in therapy when that same affect was powerfully experienced (often to the child's amazement). The therapist makes space for the child in her/his mind, something that Winnicott reported that "good enough" mothers do. In countless interactions the child expects rejection, but the therapist responds with acceptance. The child expects judgment, the therapist responds with understanding. The enraged child anticipates a punitive response, the therapist responds with tolerance. In the course of psychotherapy with children, innumerable transactions between child and therapist result in an emotionally corrective, relational healing experience.

What happens when therapists respond in the expected way? The short answer is resistance (hiding). The child is well versed in responses that reflect judgment, punishment, rejection, and hostility. Most therapists will not succeed with a child they respond to in the usual way, whether via power struggles, lecturing, or criticism expressed verbally or, even more commonly, by body language, particularly facial expressions and tone of voice. As all experienced child therapists know, children are not easily fooled. They have an uncanny ability to discern whether the therapist is genuinely seeking or whether they (children) need to hide.

CONCLUSION

While there is no doubt that some children are adamantly opposed to therapy from the outset, this chapter resists the concept of resistance in child therapy. The therapy process is conceptualized partially as a sophisticated version of hide-and-seek. The child in hiding depends on a determined seeker in order to be "found." This dynamic is a part of what play reveals consciously and often unconsciously in the therapy session. In the end, the wisdom emanating from the classic "hide-and-seek" of childhood can't be ignored. What child in hiding doesn't ultimately want to be found?

FIVE RECOMMENDED PRACTICES

1. Never assume that you know what the child thinks or feels. Children are strongly offended by such assumptions and will clam up.

2. Never convey a judgmental attitude by verbalization or nonverbal communication. Youth will read it every time, no matter how hard you try to hide it, and they will not feel safe with you and will clam up. The nonverbal communication can best be monitored by clients' immediate reactions and sometimes they will tell us directly how much they are offended by our judgmental attitudes.

3. Never compare your hardships with the client's and never tell the child, "When I was a child, . . ." The child is guaranteed to clam up and be convinced that you don't understand (and we don't).

4. The therapeutic context created must be safe, comfortable, playful, and inviting to children in order for them to be motivated to do the hard work of therapy.

5. We must do our own work either in our own therapy and/or supervision or consultation with more experienced/wiser colleagues to minimize microaggressions that will surely shut down the therapy process and to lead to clam up.

REFERENCES

Anderson, J., Martin, J., Mullen, P., Romans, S., & Herbison, P. (1993). Prevalence of childhood sexual abuse experiences in a community sample of women. *Journal of American Academy of Child and Adolescent Psychiatry, 32,* 911–919.

Bonime, W. (1989). *Collaborative psychoanalysis: Anxiety, depression, dreams, and personality change.* Rutherford, NJ: Fairleigh Dickinson University Press.

Brodsky, S. L. (2011). *Therapy with coerced and reluctant clients.* Washington, DC: American Psychological Association.

Caprioli, S., & Crenshaw, D. A. (2015). The culture of silencing child victims of sexual abuse: Implications for child witnesses in court. *Journal of Humanistic Psychology, 55,* 1–20.

Crenshaw, D. A. (2007). Play therapy with selective mutism: When Melissa speaks, everyone listens. *Play Therapy, 2*(2), 20–21.

Crenshaw, D. A. (2008). *Therapeutic engagement of children and adolescents: Play, symbol, drawing, and storytelling strategies.* Lanham, MD: Jason Aronson.

Crenshaw, D. A., & Kenny-Noziska, S. (2014). Therapeutic presence in play therapy. *International Journal of Play Therapy, 23*(1), 31–43.

Eisen, G. (1988). *Children and play in the Holocaust: Games among the shadows.* Amherst: University of Massachusetts Press.

Fleming, J. M. (1997). Prevalence of childhood sexual abuse in a community sample of Australian women. *Medical Journal of Australia, 166,* 65–68.

Fussner, A., & Crenshaw, D. A. (2008). Healing the wounds of children in a family contest. In D. A. Crenshaw (Ed.), *Child and adolescent psychotherapy: Wounded spirits and healing paths* (pp. 31–48). Lanham, MD: Jason Aronson.

Geller, S. M., & Porges, S. W. (2014). Therapeutic presence: Neurophysiological mechanisms mediating feeling safe in therapeutic relationships. *Journal of Psychotherapy Integration, 24*(3), 178–192.

Gil, E., & Crenshaw, D. A. (2015). *Termination challenges in child psychotherapy.* New York: Guilford Press.

Graybar, S. R., & Leonard, L. M. (2005). In defense of listening. *American Journal of Psychotherapy, 59*(1), 1–18.

Himelstein, S. (2013). *A mindfulness-based approach to working with high-risk adolescents.* New York: Routledge.

Lyon, T. D. (2014). Interviewing children. *Annual Review of Law and Social Science, 10,* 73–89.

Malchiodi, C. A. (1998). *Understanding children's drawings.* New York: Guilford Press.

Miller, W. R., & Rollnick, S. (1991). *Motivational interviewing: Preparing people to change addictive behavior.* New York: Guilford Press.

Nagy, P. (2010). Motivational interviewing. In M. K. Dulcan (Ed.), *Dulcan's textbook of child and adolescent psychiatry* (pp. 915–924). Arlington, VA: American Psychiatric Publishing.

Nussbaum, G. A. (2010). Impasses or development?: Understanding defiance in women with histories of childhood sexual abuse. *Issues in Psychoanalytic Psychology, 32*(1–2), 227–236.

Papp, P. (1983). *The process of change.* New York: Guilford Press.

Rogers, C. (1995). *A way of being.* New York: Houghton Mifflin.

Segal, J. (2010). The return of the absent father. In K. V. Mortensen & L. Grunbaum (Eds.), *Play and power: The EFPP book series* (pp. 115–128). London: Karnac Books.

van der Kolk, B. (2014). *The body keeps the score: Brain, mind, and body in the healing of trauma.* New York: Viking Press.

Volavkova, H. (1978). *I never saw another butterfly: Children's drawings and poems from Terezín Concentration Camp 1942–1944.* New York: Schocken Books.

Winnicott, D. H. (1965). Communicating and not communicating leading to a study of certain opposites. In *The maturational processes and the facilitating environment* (pp. 177–192). New York: International Universities Press.
Winnicott, D. W. (1951). Hate in the countertransference. *International Journal of Psychoanalysis, 30,* 69–75.

A Neurosequential Therapeutics Approach to Guided Play, Play Therapy, and Activities for Children Who Won't Talk

Richard L. Gaskill
Bruce D. Perry

Over the past century, play therapists have designed a remarkable array of theories, techniques, play therapy skills, and intervention strategies intended to help troubled children. These myriad play therapy methods largely evolved out of existing adult therapies (Gaskill & Perry, 2014). Early pioneers in children's therapy quickly recognized the poor fit between adult therapeutic strategies and the developmental limitations of children. Adaptations to accommodate children began almost immediately (Lebo, 1982). In spite of these changes, it is still common for children to fail to respond to existing play therapy strategies. Children can become exceptionally resistive to well-intentioned and badly needed therapeutic assistance. Such resistance can quickly morph into open defiance, including tantrums, withdrawal, even refusal to talk. Such events create substantial frustration for therapist, child, and family and jeopardize the therapeutic process. Often, this results from either an overestimate of the child's capacity to verbally participate in therapeutic activities or emphasizing concepts beyond the child's developmental capacity. Such expectations take the "play" out of play therapy.

In the past 20 years, new insights into the emotional, social, cognitive, and behavioral effects of developmental trauma have suggested new tools to help children affected by developmental chaos, threat, violence, and trauma. When therapists, parents, and teachers understand the children's altered functional capacity, expectations for the child become more realistic and adults are able to assist the child with developmentally suitable interventions. Employing developmentally sensitive and trauma-informed skills greatly improves the effectiveness of interventions including play therapy (Barfield, Dobson, Gaskill, & Perry, 2012; Gaskill & Perry, 2012, 2014; Hansen, 2011).

EARLY PLAY THERAPY ADAPTATIONS

Early play therapy pioneers were quick to recognize the importance of play when working with children. It was obvious that children, especially younger children, were incapable discussing their anxieties, disinterested in conversing about past experiences or memories, and attended therapy only at their parents' insistence. Consequently, many early analysts refused to treat children, choosing instead to consult with parents based on observations of the children (O'Conner, 2000). Hermine von Hug-Hellmuth was the first to consider play essential to child analysis (Lebo, 1982). By the 1920s, Anna Freud and Melanie Klein were writing extensively about play in therapy. They contended that play helped children to work through their difficulties or traumas by helping them gain insight. Klein thought play was the natural method of expression for children, as their verbal skills were insufficiently developed (Bratton & Ray, 2000; O'Conner, 2000). The use of play was a significant advancement in work with troubled children.

A second advancement in children's treatment began in the late 19th century with the expanding knowledge of child development largely due to the work of Freud, Gesell and Ilg, Piaget, Kohlberg, Vygotsky, Erikson, and others (Keil, 2000). This growing body of knowledge further increased the appreciation of the cognitive limitations and the overemphasis of verbally mediated interventions with children. Developmental researchers found young children (5 to 12 years of age) had an inadequate conceptual understanding of categories or classifications and were less able to manage multiple classification problems. These normal developmental limitations persist over long periods of time, resulting in fragmented and disorganized conceptual understanding. Such developmental immaturity renders young children heavily dependent on sensory experience rather than cognitive understanding to make sense of the world around them (Piaget, 1962; Watts-English, Fortson, Gibler, Hooper, & DeBellis, 2006). Further compounding this limited verbal and conceptual ability is the observation that children from low verbal families develop language skills even more slowly (Hart & Risley, 2003). This results in protracted immature language usage, fewer words, shorter sentences, and the consideration of fewer details than children from high verbal families (Papalia & Olds, 1979). Taken collectively, such limiting factors led Landreth (2002) to proclaim that verbally and cognitively mediated therapies are obviously problematic for the immature cognitive and language skills of children generally, but even more pronounced for children from low verbal families and maltreated children. Today, neurobiological research confirms these observations. Top-down, prefrontal-mediated treatment strategies prove effective only when individuals have mature cognitive and language skills (Lidzba, Schwilling, Grodd, Krageloh-Mann, & Wilke, 2011).

Verbally and cognitively mediated therapeutic approaches with children tend to overlook developmental limitations, the necessity for repeated sensory experiences, and the crucial role of adults in the acquisition of language and cognitive skills (McConachy, Bartlett, Biddle, & Lunken, 2013; Norton & Norton, 1997). While thinking, reasoning, and language abilities are desirable endpoints, children's immature development largely precludes their use as a medium of treatment. Clearly, as Landreth (1982, 2002) pointed out, the dynamics of expression and the vehicle for communication are different for children than for adults. He pointed out that children have substantial difficulty expressing in words how they feel or how they were affected by experiences. Landreth offered the admonition that restricting a child to verbal expression of feelings, thoughts, or experience unfairly limits communication between therapist and child. The result of these treatment adaptations further enhanced therapeutic efforts for troubled children and resulted in myriad therapeutic options attempting to help children express themselves. Even with these advancements, communication difficulties persisted. Researchers have just recently become aware of the magnitude of developmental, health, and behavioral problems—including speech and language problems—that plague maltreated children (McConachy et al., 2013).

In the 1990s, the introduction of complex imaging tools (magnetic resonance imaging, positron emission tomography, single photon emission computed tomography, and functional magnetic resonance imaging) provided opportunities to examine some of the neurodevelopmental effects of maltreatment and trauma on the developing brain. These changes included not only physical changes in brain architecture, but also dynamic processing alterations within the brain (DeBellis, 2001; Delima & Vimpani, 2011; Perry & Pollard, 1998; Perry, Pollard, Blakely, Baker, & Vigilante, 1995). With mounting evidence of the disrupted development of key neural networks following developmental adversity, the need to create developmentally sensitive and biologically informed approaches to help maltreated children becomes more apparent. To fully utilize these promising advances, play therapists must understand a few fundamental principles of brain development and recognize how developmental adversity can alter the normal developmental trajectory.

NORMAL BRAIN DEVELOPMENT

The human brain develops from the intrauterine period through young adult life. The astoundingly complex processes of neurogenesis, migration, synaptogenesis, synaptic sculpting, apoptosis, and myelination create thousands of neural networks across hundreds of brain regions. Neurodevelopment is a sequential process; the successful neural organization in one phase of development depends on adequate organization in the preceding phases. This sequential neural development progresses through a succession of sensitive periods in which the crucial neural organization in any given phase is shaped by the nature, timing, and pattern of specific experiences. The result of this complex dynamic process is the progressive maturation of the central nervous system and the autonomic nervous system.

The brain is interconnected through all of its various regions by multiple neural networks. Key regulatory networks, for example, originate in lower brain regions (brainstem and diencephalon controlling life-support and regulatory functions) and directly connect with higher brain regions (limbic and cortex mediating emotional, social, and cognitive functioning). These key neural networks (such as noradrenergic, adrenergic, serotonergic, and dopaminergic) also mediate neuroendocrine, neuroimmune, and autonomic nervous system functioning, allowing direct and indirect influence and input throughout the body (Delima & Vimpani, 2011; Perry, 2001). Due to their widespread distribution and central location to all afferent sensory input, these neural networks affect all physical, motor, social, emotional, and cognitive functioning and are key mediators of the variety of stress responses such as the "arousal" response and dissociation. These neural networks are malleable, and changes in sensitivity and reactivity can occur in response to environmental influences—including chaos, threat, and trauma.

When development is characterized by consistent, predictable challenges with attentive and attuned adult caregiving, the experiences of childhood help create a healthy, flexible, and capable stress response capacity that optimizes self-regulation and executive functioning (Perry, 2008, 2009). Caregivers are essential to teaching children this self-regulatory process. Through caregivers, children learn to maintain the balance between stimulation and calming behaviors, slowly learning to self-modulate or self-regulate. Gradually, children move from sensorial regulation by caregivers to relational regulation by caregivers to finally becoming self-regulated. As these abilities develop, children become better able to manage stimulation and are less vulnerable to the effects of excessive arousal (De Bellis, Keshavan, et al., 1999; Perry, 2008; Watts-English et al., 2006). Self-regulation has been called the cornerstone of early childhood development, cutting across all domains of behaviors (Zigler, Singer, & Bishop-Josef, 2004). Unfortunately, early childhood maltreatment is extraordinarily damaging to self-regulatory processes. The restoration and organization of self-regulation is central to treatment.

NEUROBIOLOGICAL IMPLICATIONS OF MALTREATMENT

The strength and the vulnerability of young children is the sensitivity of their developing brains to environmental input (Perry, 2008). Young children are powerfully affected by extreme, unpredictable, or uncontrollable activation of the stress response system through abuse, neglect, prenatal alcohol or drug exposure, or other untoward traumatic experiences. Such excessive and uncontrolled activation of the stress response system can result in overly sensitized and chronically aroused stress response networks (Perry, 2008; Unger & Perry, 2012). The resulting impact on brain architecture can adversely affect cognitive, emotional, behavioral, social, sensorimotor, and physical health problems (Anda et al., 2001; DeBellis et al., 1999; Delima & Vimpani, 2011; Felitti et al., 1998; Perry, 2006, 2008, 2009; Perry & Dobson, 2013; Watts-English et al., 2006). The manifestations of maltreatment are profuse, potentially involving all bodily systems, can be overwhelming, and persist throughout a lifetime (Anda et al., 2006; Watts-English et al., 2006).

Somatic and Cognitive Impacts of Trauma

Developmental trauma increases risk for a host of symptoms, physical signs, and altered functioning, including: intrusive recollections, avoidance of associated stimuli, numbing of general responsiveness, hyperarousal, hypervigilance, increased startle response, sleep difficulties, irritability, physiological hyperactivity, behavioral impulsivity, increased muscle tone, anxiety, threat-sensitive reactions, affect regulation, language disorders, fine and gross motor delays, disorganized attachment, dysphoria, attention difficulties, cognitive deficits, memory problems, and hyperactivity (De Bellis, Keshavan, et al., 1999; Delima & Vimpani, 2011; Perry et al., 1995). It is imperative that child therapists understand that two thirds of all maltreated children exhibit brainstem and diencephalic-mediated dysregulation of gastrointestinal processes, cardiac activity, blood pressure, respiration, anxiety, or hypervigilance. All of these are predictable consequences of chronic dysregulation of the stress response systems (Hopper, Spinazzola, Simpson, & van der Kolk, 2006; Perry, 2001, 2008). The specific impact of chronic developmental adversity for a child depends on multiple variables including genetics, epigenetics, intrauterine environment, early bonding experiences, history of developmental adversity, and relational buffers (Unger & Perry, 2012). It should be noted that the incidence of psychiatric disorders found in maltreated children is so prevalent that it encompasses nearly all DSM diagnoses (Perry, 2008; Perry & Dobson, 2012). Taken as a whole, maltreatment and neglect demonstrate a powerful capacity to create enduring dysfunction in multiple domains. The earlier in a child's life maltreatment occurs, the greater the risk of enduring and pervasive problems into adulthood (Perry, 2005, 2008).

Impact of Maltreatment on Language

Speech and language development interconnects with all other facets of child development, including physical, cognitive, social, and emotional domains. Each domain affects and is affected by all other domains, assuring that language development and functioning will be altered by trauma. In fact, a history of maltreatment places a child at high risk for numerous speech and language problems, including language production, articulation, language comprehension, and school readiness (McConachy et al., 2013; Watts-English et al., 2006). Watts-English et al. went on to report that children suffering from physical abuse display deficits in verbal and memory skills as well. Specifically, preschoolers displayed lower general cognitive skills, motor skills, expressive and receptive language abilities, and syntactic delays (Eigsti & Cicchetti, 2004; Watts-English et al., 2006). Likewise, Eigsti and Cicchetti reported teens as having lower language arts skills and more limited use of self-related language, lesser use of syntax, greater self-repetitions, lower verbal and full-scale IQ scores, and lower verbal declarative memory. They continued by describing maltreating mothers as speaking less to their children and with less variety in their comments, correlating with lower verbal skills. They also found maltreatment exacerbated preexisting syntactic delays leading to failures in multiple areas of language development over time. Eigsti and Cicchetti further reported that maltreatment was correlated with deficits in cognitive verbal processing. Communication difficulties have also been associated with educational delays, forming meaningful attachments, and delays in development of a sense of self and others. Finally, Eigsti and Cicchetti found emotional, social, and cognitive delays further exacerbated existing language problems. Without remediation these problems were likely to persist into adulthood, even though evidence suggested the negative effects may be reversible with early detection and intervention (Watts-English et al., 2006). Unmistakably, speech and language difficulties hinder therapeutic work with maltreated children. Language deficits can impede formation of the therapeutic relationship, hinder communication of important therapeutic concepts, and decrease the effectiveness of language-mediated interventions. Cortically mediated strategies (top down or verbally facilitated) are problematic with young children generally and specifically with children displaying serious language problems stemming from traumatic or neglectful experiences. Left untreated, these language problems persist, hindering treatment and affecting clients' daily lives.

Currently, there is a dearth of evidence-based treatment options for complex trauma in children (Malchiodi, 2008). Most evidence-based therapies (psychodynamic, experiential, and cognitive-behavioral therapy-based play therapies) that emphasize understanding, emotional processing, insight, and problem solving pay scant attention to disturbed autonomic physical sensation and preprogramed physical actions rooted in dysregulated neural networks originating in low brain areas (brainstem [BS] and diencephalon [DE]). Traditional therapies work well with cognitive and emotional (cortically and limbically mediated) trauma issues when the core regulatory neural networks (e.g., norepinephrine [NE], serotonin, dopamine [DA] originating in the lower areas of the brain) are well organized and integrated (Perry, 2006; van der Kolk, 2004, 2006). However, affective neuroscience (Panksepp, 2008; Panksepp & Bevin, 2012) points out that thoughts are not always stronger than affects and cognitive interventions do not work well with serious pathologies. As most play therapists have observed, when affect maintains the upper hand, the "talking cure" is apt to fail, as interpretive methods are ineffective with primal passions. The reality is that children suffering from complex trauma issues will first need interventions to organize and regulate overly sensitized lower-originating neural networks and, later, interventions targeting cortically originating networks. These cortically targeted cognitive interventions will help integrate memories and experiences into a verbally coherent, understandable, and manageable set of recollections; yet this cannot occur if the child (or adult) is too dysregulated to access or effectively use his or her cortical systems.

The multiple consequences of early child maltreatment call for early identification and intervention with strategies that are effective to children with poorly developed cognitive and verbal abilities. Symptoms mediated through the regulatory neural networks originating in lower brain regions are far less responsive to treatment interventions using verbal, logical, rational, or even emotionally expressive treatment modalities. This is also true of play therapy strategies utilizing these methodologies. van der Kolk (2004) pointed out that traumatized individuals show little activity in the left hemisphere, particularly in language areas, resulting in decreased capacity for planning and analyzing while displaying excessive activity in the right limbic hemisphere, suggesting excessive emotional experience, but no ability to communicate it or understand it. Not surprisingly, such individuals respond poorly to cognitive, verbal, and multimodal treatment designs due to their self-regulatory deficits and language-based limitations.

Symptoms arising from dysregulated neural networks of the BS and DE respond best to treatments focused on the child's regulatory deficits, reserving cortical interventions for when the child is less reactive and impulsive (i.e., regulated). The developmentally limited verbal and cognitive abilities of children further diminished by maltreatment call for bottom-up treatment strategies, with the highest probability of providing the patterns of activation likely to organize and reorganize the regulatory neural networks of the BS and DE. Only after bottom-up modalities (primary sensory, somatic, movement, rhythmic) help establish basic homeostatic stability will top-down treatments such as insight, reflection, trauma integration, narrative development, social development, or affect enhancement be effective (Kliem & Jones, 2008; Perry, 2008, 2009). Of foremost importance in the treatment of early childhood trauma is establishing basic state regulation and maintaining appropriate relational, language, and cognitive expectations for the child's developmental age rather than chronological age. The challenge becomes integrating a neurodevelopmentally informed perspective into play therapy and children's therapy generally (Gaskill & Perry, 2012, 2014).

PLAY, PLAY THERAPY, AND PLAY ACTIVITIES GUIDED BY THE NEUROSEQUENTIAL MODEL OF THERAPEUTICS

Once state regulation and healthy homeostasis have been established, cortically mediated cognitive-behavioral treatments will be more effective (see Perry & Dobson, 2013; Perry & Hambrick, 2008). With many young maltreated children, this may require developing healthy homeostasis for the first time. Using a bottom up methodology of trauma-informed care, establishing a sense of safety and self-regulation must precede insight, reflection, trauma integration, emotional processing, relational engagement, or positive affect enhancement, as these are mediated through cortical and limbic areas and predicated on regulatory competence to succeed (Cook et al., 2005).

Perry (2008) outlined four core elements in positive developmental experiences rooted in neurobiological processes (e.g., neuroplasticity) and essential to healthy neural development. Healthy development, he said, was maximized by experiences that were relevant or developmentally matched to the child's current stage of growth. Second, he stated experiences should be repetitive and patterned, meaning repeated in similar ways over time. Third, he asserted successful positive development occurred when the child was in a safe, nurturing relationship with caregivers. Last, Perry spoke of the importance of the natural rhythms of positive entrainment, the neurobiological process of synchronization of the child and adult. These core elements, Perry claimed, were developmentally imperative to all children, including the treatment of children suffering from abuse. Trauma-informed interventions that adhere to these fundamental neurobiological principles are more likely to provide optimal outcomes. A number of studies have demonstrated the effectiveness of neurodevelopmentally informed approaches over talk therapies or pharmacological approaches in reducing core trauma symptoms and promoting healthy social–emotional development (Barfield et al., 2011; Hansen, 2011; Miranda, Arthur, Mahoney, & Perry, 1998; Miranda, Schilick, Dobson, Hogan, & Perry, 1999; van der Kolk et al., 2007)

Core Element 1: Relevant

A basic tenet of neuroplasticity is "specificity"—basically, that the neural network you wish to change (either during development or later in life) must be the target of patterned, repetitive activation. Therefore, in approaching a child following complex trauma, the interventions need to provide appropriate "activation" for the neural systems that are either undeveloped or poorly organized. Hence, "trauma-informed" interventions must be matched (and sequenced) to the neural networks and brain areas that have been altered by the developmental neglect and trauma. This entails activation of the brain region mediating the symptomatology, promoting organization of that region and between regions, as well as fostering more mature functioning. To accomplish this treatment must target the lowest disorganized brain region first. The principle of

working from the "bottom up" is predicated on the hierarchical principle of brain development (mastery of lower levels first). In addition, since
internal or external sensory input is processed in lower brain regions
before transmission to upper brain regions, it is important that these
lower areas function properly. When lower brain regions are functionally disorganized and poorly integrated with higher brain regions, neural input will be defectively processed, effectively corrupting the ability
of higher centers to accurately interpret, process, and act on the information. This is reminiscent of the old computer adage, "garbage in equals
garbage out." The "bottom-up" approach is often regressive in the sense
that the low brain must have correcting experiences before higher brain
regions can function well. In addition, given that neural networks originating in lower areas tend to be less "plastic" than cortical networks,
bottom-up treatments require a consistently patterned and repetitive
treatment protocol over many treatment presentations (discussed in
Core Element 2). Last, regulatory neural networks of the BS and DE
process store and act on incoming input from the body (e.g., enterocep-
tion) and outside world in a "precortical" manner, outside conscious
awareness, verbal understanding, insight, or logic. These facts seriously
hamper verbal therapies' ability to be effective when the child is dysregulated since these therapeutic approaches are based on awareness,
conscious thought, and verbal communication. While cortical control of
BS and DE originating neural networks is possible in a well-organized,
functional, and integrated brain, such control is severely compromised
by disorganizing effects of early childhood trauma. Successful treatment will require establishing body regulation, decreased arousal, and
establishing healthy homeostasis. Once this is established, "top-down"
approaches, such as understanding what has happened, developing one's
personal narrative, and working on esteem and personal value issues,
will be effective. Since the low brain does not respond to language or
logic, the methods to achieve the early stages of treatment become paramount.

Somatosensory Focus

When symptomatology suggests poor regulation of core body functions,
over-/underarousal, impulsivity, sleep problems, attention difficulties, or
irregularities in sensory perception, the initial focus of treatment should
be the BS- and DE-originating neural networks. Children requiring
primary somatosensory interventions are likely are to display frequent
sensory misperceptions, appetite, feeding, or metabolism problems,
persistent somatic or visceral dysregulation, fine or gross motor movement or balance impairment, sleep problems, or endocrine issues. Such

anomalies will be in excess of normal for the developmental age. The treatment protocol will emphasize somatosensory experiences, self-regulation, and movement interventions, all of which provide the appropriate nature and pattern of activation to help these lower networks change. Language, reasoning, logic, and understanding are de-emphasized in favor of core regulatory functions. The somatosensory activities must be carried out in a richly positive relational context (Core Element 3) as the activity itself is insufficient for positive developmental growth and neural organization.

Sensory activities must be planned and scheduled at specific times each day for short periods of about 10 to 15 minutes. Pick activities the child will enjoy, as children will not repeat those that are unrewarding. The activity, environment, and method may need to modified periodically to keep them fresh, attractive, and fun. Never force the child into an activity if he or she is uncomfortable with it. Take baby steps if the child is uncomfortable. Find safe ways for the child to engage in and experience the activity. Let the child lead, but supervise the activity to prevent overstimulation (Kranowitz & Newman, 2010).

At this stage, introduce soothing and calming play or play activities such as: gentle touches, swinging in a swing/glider, using a rocking chair, putting lotion on boo-boos, face painting, listening to music, natural sounds, hugs, stroking, massage, use of comforters, pillows, stuffed animals, fidgets, sensory bags, wiggle cushions, reading stories, poetry, rhyming songs, playing with clay, sand, or texture boxes with many textures to feel. Also effective are games or active play with piggyback rides, swings, exercise equipment, bean bags, playing catch, or running an obstacle course. The list of activities is only limited by one's imagination. The object is to sense with one's body, to feel opposites (fast/slow, calm/excited, energized/tired, and so on), and experience calmness, quiescence, pleasure, and relaxation with a trusted caregiver.

Relational/Affective Focus

The social or relational networks in the limbic system are involved in affective experience and interpretation of affective stimuli, including relational behavior, a sense of attunement, and a sense of reward and pleasure. Understanding the emotional experiences of others and responding appropriately with empathy is important aspect of this region, as is forming lasting relationships, taking turns, sharing, and psychosocial development. These social and emotional functions are both semiconscious and conscious, and can be expressed behaviorally as well as verbally. However, the affective experiences are not associated with logic, planning, or reason. Children struggling with affective and relational difficulties may not display the normal range of emotion, do not regulate their emotions well, have difficult relationships with others, and feel little pleasure or reward from normal experience. They may also display little age-appropriate empathy, have difficulty delaying gratification, or may have learning or memory difficulties.

Treatment protocols for difficulties in these functions focus on emotional processing, not cognitive functions such as abstraction, conceptual understanding, problem solving, or planning. The primary focus is empathy, attachment, attunement, and positive emotions related to interpersonal relationships. The therapist must emphasize face-to-face gaze, eye-to-eye contact, matching facial expression, matching tone of voice, and using reflective responses. Also effective are play and play activities, such as singing, music, enjoyable social activities, playing with a pet, telling stories, special handshakes, playing with stacking blocks, Legos, or manipulatives, games that allow taking turns, playing with a cardboard box maze, playing social games (Red Light, Green Light; Mother, May I; Simon Says; Duck, Duck, Goose; Sorry!; Candyland), dramatic play, reading stories of social experiences (Aesop's fables, Annie's Stories, Berenstain Bears), puppet plays, family rituals, cooperation games, memory games, and sociodramatic play.

Cognitive Focus

Cognitive methodologies (cortically mediated) are most appropriate when the networks of the lower areas (BS, DE) are more functional. Cognitive strategies include thinking (understanding, labeling, categorizing, conceptualizing), creativity, planning, and problem-solving strategies. The neocortex carries out our most highly evolved mental activities. It allows us to be most human and humane (Szalavitz & Perry, 2010), but it is the last brain region to mature. The cortex reprocesses information provided by lower regions and is responsible for analyzing and understanding and, when necessary, acting on the information and responses coming from lower regions. The cortex allows us to integrate, organize, classify, order, and manipulate multiple sensory stimuli into unified concepts, such as relationships between time, space, and matter, as well as understand ourselves and others. Our highest moral, ethical, and spiritual thoughts come from this region. Under the best circumstances, this region is capable of modulating and regulating the neural networks of the lower brain (this is basically "executive functioning"), but the cortex can be overwhelmed, disorganized, or even silenced by the incoming input of a reactive and dysregulated set of neural networks from the BS and DE. Trauma-related manifestations of impaired cortical development or functioning may include communication disorders, understanding causality, motivation, academic problems, conservation of matter, ordering events, classifying, forming hypothesis, problem solving, or moral and ethical thinking.

Treatment now focuses on cognitive, behavioral, language, and insight-oriented interventions. Most therapeutic modalities fit here as long as they are within the child's developmental level. Unfortunately, too many professionals begin here without attending to the dysregulated networks of the BS/DE. The tacit assumption is that all brain functioning arises from the cortical structures. Interventions that might be considered cortically targeted are play therapy, bibliotherapies, behavioral management, individual talk and family therapies, storytelling games, books, stories, chess, checkers, Battleship, Clue, and Concentration, as well as various therapeutic games. The performing arts and other expressive mediums become much more powerful, as do discussion about morality, values, and spirituality.

Core Element 2: Repetitive

As stated earlier, the neural networks of the BS/DE require very specific forms and patterns of activation to change and, in general, are "harder" to change than cortical networks.

A key challenge is determining the "dosing" of somatosensory targeted interventions—how much, for how long, and how many times a day? Research on implicit learning and in occupational therapy settings dealing with unconscious learning and precortical neural networks may provide some clues. Coh, Jovanovic-Golubouic, and Baltic (2004) examined the difference between learning a motor skill at an explicit level (conscious and intentional) and learning the motor action at an implicit level (unconscious and automatic). The results suggested that performing an action consciously, but awkwardly, took approximately 30 hours of practice. To perform the same action unconsciously and with precision required as many as 50,000 practice episodes. A similar learning pattern was found in a preschool population of children with visual–motor integration and performance problems. Golos, Sarid, Weil, and Weintraub (2011) reported improvement in visual–motor performance after approximately 8 months of weekly practice. Both of these studies suggest that "deep" learning, involving neural networks of the lower areas of the brain, takes many episodes. Fortunately, this is possible when one considers that for reorganizing the stress response networks and the neural systems most affected by maltreatment, a therapeutic "episode" may be merely seconds of the appropriate interaction when this episode is with an attentive, attuned, and nurturing adult. In any given positive interaction, therefore, of say, 10 minutes, dozens of "doses" of therapeutic repetition are possible. This reality suggests that progress will be quicker if parents, teachers, and therapists all work together to form a consistent therapeutic web supporting positive change.

Finally, routines and rituals are vital components of the repetitive and patterned core element. Routines and rituals provide familiar and reinforcing stimulation, creating a safe and predictable set of stimuli for the child. Since the brain's lower neural networks assess incoming stimuli for similarities to prior experiences, it is not surprising that routine and rituals provide sensory input that the world is consistent and predictable. Landreth (2002) captured this perfectly when he said that consistency equals predictability and predictability equals security. In addition, a predictable pattern of social routines communicates unity, connectedness, and permanency in the relationship. Therapists must be aware of and sensitive to the rituals children create in the lobby, playroom, and home, encouraging caregivers to honor these rituals as a way of creating a sense of safety. Children do not develop healthily when they are in a constant state of threat. Rituals and routines are a time-honored way that adults communicate to children I am here, I hear you, I understand, and I care (Landreth, 2002).

Core Element 3: Relational

Humans are an interdependent, relational species. Trauma-informed work must be carried out in a warm, positive, relational context; this is a neurobiological necessity if the goal is health, growth, and development. We survive because we have the capacity to form rewarding, nurturing, loving, and enduring relationships (Szalavitz & Perry, 2010). Human beings desire and seek positive relationships from the first moments of life and continue to seek proximity to those relationships throughout life. Recent research suggests that positive emotions (warmth expressed through kind words, touch, smiles, and laughter) contribute to ideal neural functioning with optimal levels of neurogenesis and neuroplasticity (Ponkanen & Hietanen, 2012). These positive emotions are communicated nonverbally by the whole body, but the face and eyes are the predominant medium of social communication (Schilbach, Eickhoff, Mojzisch, & Vogeley, 2008). Displaying positive social emotions, especially smiling and laughter, are consistently interpreted as trustworthy, familiar, and attractive (Nelson, & Jeste, 2008; Niedenthal, Mermillod, Maringer, & Hess, 2010; O'Doherty et al., 2003; Ponkanen & Hietanen, 2012). Negative emotions (frowns or scowls), on the other hand, lead to protective responses in observers, suppressing neurogenesis, possibly an attempt to limit the impact of negative stimuli. Human beings require relational reward and safety to make positive developmental gains, both socially and intellectually. It is not surprising that human beings seek out and thrive in positive social environments. Given our predisposition for seeking out positive relationships, it makes sense that the therapist–client alliance is one of the most predictive measures therapy outcomes (Shirk & Karver, 2011). Emphasizing the use of social interactional behaviors is fundamental to relationship building and successful treatment.

A final relational aspect central to successful treatment is the ratio of adults to children. During the "tender years" of early childhood, the ratio of adults to children is ideally very low, often one to one. This close relationship is necessary for a child's survival. Even older children with developmental delays will require lower adult-to-child ratios than their chronological age would suggest. We have found this to be one of the most important treatment variables contributing to successful intervention, yet this is one of the most difficult principles for adults to understand about older maltreated children. Success often depends on the opportunity to practice a new skills within a warm, supportive, patient, positive relationship with an adult (scaffolding) until the new skill has been mastered. Once this happens, the skill is much more likely to appear in other environments.

Core Element 4: Rhythm

The final core element is rhythm, which Perry (2006, 2008) described as resonating with the neural patterns of positive entrainment. This element is the driver of positive change and is firmly positioned on the foundational aspects of the other three core elements. The culmination of these core elements is truly a remarkable process of organizing and integrating the profoundly complex neural networks of the human brain. As the adult meets the child's basic needs in a calm, open, emotionally nurturing state, a harmonic joining of the two brains occurs. This synchronous relationship includes face-to-face gaze and eye-to-eye contact between parent and child. In this state the right cortex, EEGs, heart waves, and hormonal systems synchronize. Early childhood experts refer to this as co-regulation, a core element in teaching children how to self-regulate later in life. Children who lack this experience have difficulty forming healthy attachments later in life (Panksepp & Bevin, 2012). This remarkable process involves many systems in the brain, including several "mirror neuron" systems (Rizzolatti, 2005). Specialized motor neurons in the temporal parietal area of the brain, for example, mimic the motor and emotional behavior observed in others. This is part of the complex neurobiological mechanisms through which we understand the actions, intentions, and emotions of others (Pfeifer, Iacoboni, Mazziotta, & Dapretto, 2008). Furthermore, this process engenders a genuineness of social interactions, positive emotional responses, and the affective mood displayed (Leslie, Johnson-Frey, & Grafton, 2004). Leslie et al. found that conscious control of facial musculature during imitation activated different neural systems than when it happened automatically (genuinely). This suggests that conscious imitation is analogous to masking one's intentions rather than an empathic response. Children commonly observe and imitate emotional faces of others, beginning by 10 weeks of age, and are good judges of genuineness and authenticity (Pfeifer et al., 2008). Genuine empathy cannot easily be faked. The neurobiologically mediated "contagion" of the human brain provides a very specialized nonverbal method of teaching and learning about others. The ability to become genuinely attuned with others is an essential skill for all adults working with children.

The Neurosequential Model of Therapeutics™ (NMT) is a developmentally sensitive, trauma-informed approach to clinical problem solving. It allows the clinician to gather a systematic developmental history of both adversity and resilience-related factors. In addition, an assessment of current functioning is converted into a heuristic of the client's "brain" functioning. This "Brain Map" allows the clinician to identify the specific systems and areas of the brain that the therapeutic process should target. This allows the clinician to select and sequence therapeutic, educational, and enrichment experiences that will plausibly provide the nature, pattern, and timing of experience required to help the child move toward a healthier developmental trajectory. The case below is an example of putting the principles outlined above into practice.

CASE EXAMPLE

Billy is a 7-year-old Caucasian boy; while he is a fictitious child, his history and problems represent a composite derived from actual children with serious and complex histories of developmental trauma and neglect. He is a quiet child and seems generally agreeable with adult requests unless he is upset. Billy has a pleasant smile that he displays most of the time until he tantrums. He gets along best with his adoptive mother, as his adoptive father is much more easily frustrated with his actions. The father sees Billy as needing to "just grow up" and pressures him as if this is within is ability to do so, "if he would only try."

Billy's biological parents struggled with drug abuse and dependence before and during his intrauterine period. Both parents continued to use street drugs after Billy was born. His parents were chronically unemployed or underemployed and frequently engaged minor criminal behavior such as shoplifting, petty theft, and minor drug dealing to support their own use. Billy's conception was an accident, and it is not clear the parents were ever married. His parents could not maintain a stable home and often stayed in homeless shelters during the pregnancy. Billy was born prematurely as a result of the mother's drug use and spent the first week after delivery in a neonatal ICU. He did well and was placed in emergency foster care shortly after dismissal, as his parents had no home and no way to care for him upon discharge.

In the first few months after his birth, Billy's mother and father agreed to a reintegration plan, but continued drug use, criminal behavior, and failed to keep visits with Billy. When they did keep visitation, it was observed that his mother's parenting skills were poor, usually frustrating the baby, prompting the mother to hand him back to the visitation supervisor. The father was totally disengaged. Billy continued in foster care and was moved to a long-term foster home. Ultimately, his parents relinquished their parental rights within the first year of his life. The parent's unstable relationship persisted until they finally drifted apart.

Between 1 and 2 years, Billy was moved twice to new foster homes. He was a fussy baby and toddler, according to the foster care reports. The moves were prompted by the difficulty in caring for him and the foster parents' having no intentions of adopting him. He did not accept comforting well and did not seem to seek out his caregivers when hurt, hungry, or tired. At age 2½ he was placed with his fourth foster family, who eventually adopted him by age 4. This became Billy's first permanent placement. At first, the adoptive parents reported things went fairly well after an "adjustment phase." His performance in preschool and kindergarten was average, with occasional tantrums noted. Teachers and parents noted he had difficulty sitting still or staying seated, and his language skills were weak so he often did not understand what he was told and understanding him was difficult. He preferred to wander around the classroom or home. Parents and teachers reported having to keep an eye on him or he would wander off.

By age 3, his adoptive parents complained of sneaky behavior. His adoptive father struggled to accept the idea he could not discipline Billy out of the negative behaviors. These confrontations increasingly led to tantrums and destructive rages from Billy. By age 6, the parents reported that Billy lied over senseless things, and was stealing worthless objects and hiding them in his bedroom. He would hoard food and frequently wandered off. Billy began to threaten his family when they did not get him what he wanted, and he frequently hid from them. He still occasionally wet the bed, but hid his underwear. His parents were divided over how to handle him and agreed to seek therapy.

Upon intake it was learned that Billy had previously been diagnosed

as having attention-deficit/hyperactivity disorder (ADHD) by his pedia-
trician and had trouble going to sleep, often resisting going to bed. He
was on medications to help him sleep and to focus, but the medications
were seen as minimally helpful. Once asleep, he slept through the night,
even when he wet the bed. He was reported as always hungry and asking to be fed. Despite his persistent begging for food, he was of normal
weight and height. His foster parents generally fed him, believing he
was hungry since he was not overweight. Billy was prone to tantrums,
but they seemed to most likely to occur when he was prevented from
withdrawing or thwarted in getting what he wanted. His tantrums were
occasionally destructive.

Billy seemed to experience reward, as he would smile and show
excitement when he was in a good mood. He displayed empathetic
responses to animals, especially the family dog. He would pet and talk
to the dog often, but was occasionally too rough with him.

Billy's memory seemed to work well for the things important to
him, making average grades in school, yet his adoptive mother complained that he did not seem to learn from mistakes. Billy had continued
trouble expressing himself verbally, especially regarding affective experiences, so he more often expressed his emotions nonverbally. He did not
seem able to communicate his intent, meaning, or purpose well. He was
more able to express what he wanted or what he did not want in simple
declarative statements, without underlying meaning. Finally, Billy was
frequently unable to control himself once he became frustrated. He was
easily overwhelmed by events and lost the ability to cortically modulate
his impulses quickly.

Treatment with Billy and his family involved taking a detailed developmental and social history, as well as an assessment and treatment plan
using the NMT. The number of adverse events in the child's life suggested
a high-risk environment during his intrauterine period into early childhood. His circumstance improved after adoption, but his new family
struggled to understand his behavior, so moderate relational risk continued. Billy suffered from difficulties with sleep, appetite/feeding, metabolism, primary sensory integration, attention, visceral systems problems,
as well as dissociative reactions to stressful events. At the relational level
(limbic), Billy seemed to have affect regulation issues/tantrums, relational attachment and attunement difficulties, as well as some memory
problems. All of these problems likely interfered with his cognitive functions, which were complicated by his difficulty with verbal comprehension and expression.

The first stage of treatment was to visit with his adoptive parents and
school personnel to help them understand Billy's neurodevelopmental
difficulties and how these played out in his daily life. His NMT-derived

"Brain Map" (see Figure 3.1) was a visual aid to this discussion. As can be seen in Figure 3.1, Billy's functional capabilities (the darker the shade of gray in a specific brain region, the more underdeveloped/disorganized that region is compared to an age-typical child) are considerably below those of a typical 6- to 7-year-old. The substance abuse and early chaos in his life left Billy developmentally immature and neurologically less organized than his age mates. In fact, his behavior would be expected to be that of a much younger child based his current level of brain organization. Billy's ability to regulate the most fundamental bodily systems (heart rate, metabolism, autonomic arousal, and attention) were less well developed than a newborn child. This observation explained his overeating, hoarding, lack of focus, and tantrums. In addition, higher-level brain systems were also poorly developed, leading to relational problems with others, affective lability, conceptual problems, and ultimately his academic difficulty. His parents needed to understand that his behavior was the result of developmental immaturity and sensitized stress response systems, and that treatment and parenting would have to be consistent with his functional development, not his chronological age. This became increasingly clear when his sensory integration, self-regulation, relational, and cognitive functional domains were compared to age-typical children (see Figure 3.2). Billy's neurobiological development remained seriously immature compared to his age mates, which helped the adults in his life understand that he was not willfully disobedient and refusing to "grow up" or being deliberately disrespectful to his parents. Rather, he was doing the best he could with poorly organized, immature, and overly reactive neural systems. Functionally, Billy was not 7 years old, and expectations for him needed to be lowered to be in sync with his neurodevelopmental functioning. By understanding these issues, it was hoped we could decrease the negative judgements about the meaning of his behavior and eliminate seeing his behavior as a personal affront to his parents (especially his father). This was an attempt to move the parent–child relationship to a more positive and rewarding position, so the parents could recognize and celebrate each small success Billy made.

For the first 2 months, a planned schedule of daily play with Mom or Dad was set up. The objective was to teach basic child parent relationship therapy (CPRT; Landreth & Bratton, 2006) concepts of letting the child lead, parent facilitation of play, and both genuinely enjoying the playtime. The parents were instructed to work for the sparkle in the child's eyes and to play at a time and place that would require few limits to be set. The object was to have fun. Therapy for Billy consisted of weekly visits that were used to support and consult with the parents and the initial relationship building between Billy and the therapist. At

Client (6 years, 0 months)   **Report Date: 1/31/2016**

4	5	4	4	5	4
5	7	7	5	5	6
6	5	9	7	7	7
	8	7	6	7	
	7	4	5	6	
		10	4		
		7	9		
		4	4		

Age Typical—6 to 7

7	7	7	7	7	7
9	10	9	7	7	8
8	9	10	10	8	10
	10	9	9	10	
	9	11	10	8	
		12	10		
		12	12		
		11	12		

Functional Item Key

ABST (31)	MATH (29)	PERF (27)	MOD (28)	VERB (30)	VAL (32)
SPEECH (25)	COMM (23)	SSI (21)	TIME (22)	SELF (24)	CCOG (26)
REL (19)	ATTU (17)	REW (15)	AFF (16)	SEX (18)	MEM (20)
	NE (13)	DISS (11)	ARS (12)	PSI (14)	
	FMS (9)	FEED (7)	SLP (8)	LMF (10)	
		SSG (5)	ATTN (6)		
		MET (3)	EEOM (4)		
		CV (1)	ANS (2)		

Functional Brain Map Value Key

Developmental
Functional

12	DEVELOPED
11	TYPICAL RANGE
10	
9	EPISODIC/EMERGING
8	MILD Compromise
7	
6	PRECURSOR CAPACITY
5	MODERATE Dysfunction
4	
3	UNDEVELOPED
2	SEVERE Dysfunction
1	

FIGURE 3.1. Functional brain map and key. Copyright © Bruce D. Perry MD, PhD, and The Child Trauma Academy, 2009–2013. All rights reserved. A color version of this figure is available at www.guilford.com/p/malchiodi7.

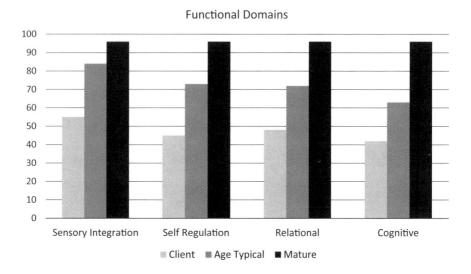

Functional Domains

FIGURE 3.2. Functional domains. Copyright © Bruce D. Perry MD, PhD, and The Child Trauma Academy, 2009–2013. All rights reserved.

this point, he did not want his parents involved in his play. Billy did not like playing in the play therapy room much at all. Instead, he was more comfortable outside wandering around the mental health center's 6-acre campus. His play was disorganized, with little or no sequencing of play themes. Largely, we wandered over the property, through the weeds into the dry creek, and caught toads and crickets. Billy was most happy doing this and seldom spoke to me. My role was to follow him around and support his play, helping him solve small problems such as how to keep our collection of pine cones, rocks, sticks, and bugs, or protecting him from stinging insects. His play was very sensory oriented and toddler-like. He mixed sticks in the mud and smeared mud, sand, sticks, grass, leaves, pine cones, water into a messy mush. A routine evolved very quickly: he and I would play outside, Billy would take off, and I would follow, supporting his efforts, and he would boss me around as if I were his servant. Billy would ask for nearly everything we came across, although nothing of any real value (Post-it notes, paper clips, small trinkets, or food). Near the end of our sessions he would tell me he was hungry. We would then go to the kitchen and have a snack of crackers, cereal, or chocolate milk before he left.

By the end of the second month, Billy was smiling more with me and beginning to engage with some comments and eye contact when he talked or smiled; occasionally he giggled or laughed. I was still a tool for him to use to meet his needs, but we had a relationship where he counted on me to help meet his needs. His play now had short, simple themes much like a preschooler. His play with his parents was similar to his play with me, and he now wanted them to play with him in the playroom on occasion. His behavior was still a problem at school, as his immaturity did not allow him to function at age-appropriate levels, but there were fewer problems that perplexed the school. At this point, we arranged for him to play with or care for puppies and kittens. This was done under supervision, with modeling and discussions about the nature of babies, whether human, canine, or feline. He learned how the animals signaled their desire for nurturing or play and how they responded to his voice, touches, and actions. Billy seemed to make good contact with the animals, talking to them and touching them gently. He enjoyed watching them seek him out.

From the third month through the sixth month Billy began engaging more physically with his parents. He was now roughhousing some with his father and playing short games with his mother. School was going better, but age-appropriate demands were still difficult for him. The school still struggled occasionally to find alternative methods of dealing with him. Billy had started some simple show-and-tell behavior with his parents and was now engaging in short interactive games like hide and seek. He was still playing with his parents at home daily. They were now allowing their playtimes to last longer, as Billy did not want to stop as soon as he had earlier. We were still unable to have family therapy with conversations about family issues. When we tried, Billy would quickly deteriorate and begin to ignore his parents, therapist, or teacher. His interactions with adults still needed to be primarily positive, as he could not handle any hint of a negative experience. He occasionally spoke of his adoptive parents as his "forever family" and was beginning to sit close to them, often with his legs across their laps. Billy's parents were gaining insights about managing his tantrums and were increasingly able to repair the relationship with more empathy and less irritation after his tantrums.

From 6 to 12 months Billy's parents continued to work at understanding his developmental age versus chronological age, accepting his regressions and using reflective listening. They continued to marvel at how much structure, routine, and patterned behavior he really needed to establish a sense of safety. He rarely wanted to play alone with me, but rather preferred his family. His play themes were becoming richer in metaphorical issues, which the parents began to understand and wanted to discuss with me. They were gaining insight into his struggles and were able to respond to him empathically with their actions and their words.

CONCLUSION

Children's therapy and play therapy have evolved significantly over the past century. Many of the improvements were the result of failed therapeutic efforts resulting in resistance to treatment. We have moved from attempting to use adult therapeutic models with children to understanding play as their natural medium, that their language skills and cognitive abilities are developmentally immature and often delayed by maltreatment, and their need for repeated sensory experiences. These incremental improvements have taught us that young children as well as maltreated children are not immediately ready for verbally mediated insight therapies. "Top-down" prefrontal-mediated treatment strategies are most affective when the client processes mature cognitive and language skills. Clear thinking, reasoning, planning, understanding, and verbal skills are desirable, but the developmental immaturity of children precludes their use, especially for children suffering from complex trauma.

Neurobiological research supports these adaptations to children's treatment and further teaches us that children's therapy must follow a developmental sequence based on functional behavior, not chronological age. Perry (2006) described this sequence as regulate, relate, and reason. Regulation becomes the first sequential step. This "trauma-informed" approach is accomplished through repeated somatosensory and movement activities, routines, rituals, soothing or calming activities, and play activities that are regulating though a richly positive interpersonal relationship. The aim at this stage is to establish body regulation, decrease arousal, and establish healthy homeostasis. Until a child is physically and emotionally settled he or she is unable to relate to others successfully. Relating to the child becomes the next step. Positive social interactional behavior is fundamental to successful treatment. Positive development for children relies on being able to practice new skills in a safe, warm, supportive, patient, positive relationship with an adult until the skill is mastered. In fact, we now know that positive emotional environments are necessary for optimal neural functioning and development. Positive emotional engagement is the supportive structure needed to learn new behaviors. Reason is the final step in the treatment process. Once children are calm and experience the safe support of a relationship, they are finally capable thinking, reasoning, and learning at their fullest potential. All three sequential steps are required for optimal physical, social–emotional, and cognitive development for all children, as well as the healing of a maltreated child.

FIVE RECOMMENDED PRACTICES

1. Children suffering from complex trauma are powerfully affected by extreme, unpredictable, or uncontrollable activation of their stress response system, resulting in overly sensitized and chronically aroused stress response networks. The resulting impact on brain architecture can adversely affect cognition, emotional, behavioral, social, sensorimotor, and physical health problems. Manifestations of maltreatment are profuse, potentially involving all body systems, and may persist throughout life. Among this array of potential problems are language production, articulation, comprehension, verbal memory, and school readiness problems.

2. Children suffering from complex trauma issues require interventions that help organized and regulate overly sensitized lower-originating neural networks, with later interventions targeting cortically originating networks. The first phase of treatment must establish basic state regulation. Early interventions must focus on primary sensory, somatic, movement, and rhythmic activities to establish basic homeostatic functioning. Routine and family rituals also help establish a sense of predictability and safety, which are important to calming and organizing low brain regions.

3. Interventions intended to target lower-originating neural networks must be planned and scheduled multiple times each day for short periods. The frequency of the activity is more important than the length of the activity. Pick activities the child enjoys so he or she will experience them as rewarding and want to repeat them. Modify the activity, environment, and method to keep it interesting, attractive, and fun. Let the child lead, but supervise to keep the child safe and to prevent overstimulation. The number and kind of activities are limitless, but they must fulfill the prime objective to sense with one's body, feel opposites, and experience calm, quiescence, pleasure, and relaxation with a trusted caregiver.

4. Interpersonal relationships are the primary focus of any intervention. Each activity must focus on empathy, attachment, attunement, and positive emotions of interpersonal relationships. An emphasis on

(continued)

FIVE RECOMMENDED PRACTICES (*continued*)

face-to-face gaze, eye contact, matching facial expressions, matching tone of voice, and using verbal and nonverbal reflective responses are of prime importance. Take the time to establish an attuned and engaged relationship, which is vital to any intervention's success. Play therapists must communicate the message "I care," "I hear you," "I understand," and "I am here."

5. The ratio of adults to children is another critical variable to successful interventions. It is generally accepted that complex trauma creates functional immaturity in children, but the immaturity also erodes the child's ability to function at an age-appropriate level of independence. A key to successful interventions is to be sure the adult-to-child ratio is consistent with their developmental age, not their chronological age. We have found this is a critical variable predicting treatment success. The greater the immaturity of the child, the lower the adult-to-child ratio must be. Some children will require a lot of one-on-one attention to make progress.

REFERENCES

Allen, R. E., & Oliver, J. M. (1982). The effects of child maltreatment on language development. *Child Abuse and Neglect, 6,* 299–305.

Anda, R. F., Felitti, V. J., Bremner, D. J., Walker, J., Whitefield, J. D., Perry, B. D., et al. (2006). The enduring effects of childhood abuse and related experiences. *European Archives of Psychiatric and Clinical Neuroscience, 256*(3), 174–186.

Anda, R. F., Felitti, V. J., Chapman, D. P., Croft, J. B., Williamson, D. F., Santelli, J., et al. (2001). Abused boys, battered mothers, and males involved in teen pregnancy. *Pediatric, 107*(2), e19.

Barfield, S., Dobson, C., Gaskill, R., & Perry, B. D. (2011). Neurosequential model of therapeutics in a therapeutic preschool: Implications for work with children with complex neuropsychiatric problems. *International Journal of Play Therapy, 21*(1), 30–44.

Bratton, S. C., Landreth, G. L., Kellam, T., & Blackard, S. R. (2006). *Child parent relationship therapy (CPRT) treatment manual: A 10-session filial therapy model for training parents.* New York: Routledge.

Bratton, S., & Ray, D. (2000). What the research shows about play therapy. *International Journal of Play Therapy, 9*(1), 47–48.

Coh, M., Jovanovic-Golubouic, D., & Baltic, M. (2004). Motor learning in sport. *Physical Education and Sport, 2*(1), 45–59.

Cook, A., Spinazzola, J., Ford, J., Lanktree, C., Blaustein, M. B., Cloitre, M., et al. (2005). Complex trauma in children and adolescents. *Psychiatric Annals, 35*(5), 390–398.

De Bellis, M. D. (2001). Developmental traumatology: The psychobiological development of maltreated children and its implications for research, treatment, and policy. *Development and Psychopathology, 13,* 539–564.

De Bellis, M. D., Baum, A. S., Birmaher, B., Keshavean, M. S., Eccard, C. H., Boring, A. M., et al. (1999). Developmental traumatology: Part I. Biological stress systems. *Biological Psychiatry, 45*(10), 1256–1270.

De Bellis, M. D., Keshavan, M. S., Clark, D. B., Casey, B. J., Giedd, J. N., Boring, A. M., et al. (1999). Developmental traumatology: Part II. Brain development. *Biological Psychiatry, 45*(10), 1271–1284.

Delima, M. D., & Vimpani, G. (2011). The neurobiolgical effects of childhood maltreatment: An often overlooked narrative related to long term effects of early childhood trauma? *Family Matters, 89,* 42–52.

Eigsti, I. M., & Cicchetti, D. (2004). The impact of child maltreatment on expressive syntax at 60 months. *Developmental Science, 7*(1), 88–102.

Felitti, V. J., Anda, R. F., Nordenberg, D., Williamson, D. F., Spitz, A. M., & Edwards, V. (1998). Relationship of childhood abuse and household dysfunction to many of the leading causes of death in adults: Adverse Childhood Event Study. *American Journal of Preventive Medicine, 14,* 245–258.

Gaskill, R. L., & Perry, B. D. (2012). Child sexual abuse, traumatic experiences, and their impact on the developing brain. In P. Goodyear-Brown (Ed.), *Handbook of child sexual abuse: Identification, assessment, and treatment* (pp. 30–47). Hoboken, NJ: Wiley.

Gaskill, R. L., & Perry, B. D. (2014). The neurobiological power of play: Using the Neurosequential Model of Therapeutics™ to guide play in healing process. In C. Malchoidi & D. Crenshaw (Eds.), *Creative arts and play therapy for attachment trauma* (pp. 178–194). New York: Guilford Press.

Golos, A., Sarid, M., Weil, M., & Weintraub, N. (2011). Efficacy of an early intervention program for at-risk preschool boys: A two-group control study. *American Journal of Occupational Therapy, 65*(4), 400–408.

Hart, B., & Risley, T. R. (2003). The early catastrophe: The 30-million word gap by age 3. *American Educator, 27*(1), 4–9.

Hansen, L. (2011). Evaluating a sensorimotor intervention in children who have experienced complex trauma: A pilot study. *Honors Project,* Paper 151.

Hopper, J. W., Spinazzola, J., Simpson, W. B., & van der Kolk, B. A. (2006). Primary evidence of parasympathetic influence. *Journal of Psychosomatic Research, 60,* 83–90.

Keil, F. C. (2000). The origins of developmental psychology. *Journal of Cognition and Development, 1*(3), 347–357.

Kleim, J. A., & Jones, T. A. (2008). Principles of experience-dependent neural plasticity: Implications of rehabilitation after brain damage. *Journal of Speech, Language and Hearing Research, 51,* 225–239.

Kranowitz, C., & Newman J. (2010). *Growing an insyc child: Simple fun activities to help every child develop, learn, and grow.* New York: Penguin.

Landreth, G. (1982). Children communicate through play. In G. Landreth (Ed.),

Play therapy: Dynamics of the process of counseling children (pp. 45–46). Springfield, IL: Charles C Thomas.

Landreth, G. (2002). *Play therapy: Art of the relationships.* New York: Brunner-Routledge.

Landreth, G., & Bratton, S. (2006). *Child parent relationship therapy (CPRT): A 10 session filial therapy model.* New York: Routledge.

Lebo, D. (1982). The development of play as a form of therapy: From Rousseau to Rogers. In G. L. Landreth (Ed.), *Play therapy: Dynamics of the process of counseling children* (pp. 65–73). Springfield, IL: Charles C Thomas.

Leslie, K. R., Johnson-Frey, S. H., & Grafton, S. T. (2004). Functional imaging of face and hand imitation: Towards a motor theory of empathy. *NeuroImage, 24,* 601–607.

Lidzba, K., Schwilling, E., Grodd, W., Krageloh-Mann, I., & Wilke, M. (2011). Language comprehension vs. language production: Age effects on fMRI activation. *Brain and Language, 119*(1), 6–15.

Malchiodi, C. A. (2008). *Creative Interventions with traumatized children.* New York: Guilford Press.

McConachy, J., Bartlett, J., Biddle, D., & Lunken, T. (2013). *Small talk final report: Identifying communication problems in children, developing a problem identification tool.* Richmond, Australia: Berry Street, Take Two Research Project.

Miranda, L. A., Arthur, A., Mahoney, O., & Perry, B. (1998). The art of healing: The healing arts project, early childhood connection. *Journal of Music and Movement-Based Learning, 4*(4), 35–40.

Miranda, L. A., Schilick, S., Dobson, C., Hogan, L., & Perry, B. (1999). The developmental effects of brief music and movement program at a public preschool: A pilot project (Abstract). Available at *www.childtrauma.org/ctaServices/neigh_artsasp.*

Nelsen, C. A., & Jeste, S. (2008). Neurobiological perspectives on developmental psychopathology. In M. Rutter, D. Bishop, D. Pine, S. Scott, J. Stevenson, E. Taylor, et al. (Eds.), *Textbook on child and adolescent psychiatry* (5th ed., pp. 145–159). London: Blackwell.

Niedenthal, P. M., Mermillod, M., Maringer, M., & Hess, U. (2010). Simulation of smiles (SIMS) model: Embodied simulation and the meaning of facial expression. *Behavioral and Brain Science, 33*(6), 417–433.

Norton, C. C., & Norton, B. E. (1997). *Reaching children through play therapy: An experiential approach.* Denver: Publishing Cooperative.

O'Conner, K. J. (2000). *The play therapy primer* (2nd ed.). New York: Wiley.

O'Doherty, J., Winston, J., Critchley, H., Perrett, D., Burt, D. M., & Dolan, R. J. (2003). Beauty in a smile: The role of medial orbitalfrontal cortex in facial attractiveness. *Neuropsychologia, 41*(2), 147–155.

Panksepp, J. (2008). *Affective neuroscience: The foundation of human and animal emotion.* New York: Oxford University Press.

Panksepp, J., & Bevin, L. (2012). *Archeology of the mind: Neuroevolutionary origins of human emotion.* New York: Norton.

Papalia, D. E., & Olds, S. W. (1979). *A child's world: Infancy through adolescence* (2nd ed.). New York: McGraw-Hill.

Perry, B. D. (2001). The neuroarcheology of childhood treatment: The neuro-developmental costs of adverse childhood events. In K. Franey, R. Gef-fner, & R. Falconer (Eds.), *The cost of maltreatment: Who pays? We all do* (pp. 15–37). San Diego, CA: Family Violence and Sexual Assault Institute.

Perry, B. D. (2005). *Maltreatment and the developing child: How early childhood experience shapes child and culture.* The Inaugural Margaret McCain Lecture (abstracted). London, Ontario, Canada: McCain Lecture Series, Centre for Children and Families in the Justice System.

Perry, B. D. (2006). Applying principles of neurodevelopment to clinical work with maltreated and traumatized children. In N. B. Webb (Ed.), *Working with traumatized youth in child welfare* (pp. 27–52). New York: Guilford Press.

Perry, B. D. (2008). Child maltreatment: A neurodevelopmental perspective on the role of trauma and neglect in psychopathology. In T. Beachaine & S. P. Hinshaw (Eds.), *Child and adolescent psychopathology* (pp. 93–129). Hoboken, NJ: Wiley.

Perry, B. D. (2009). Examining child maltreatment through a neurodevelopmental lens: Clinical application of the Neurosequential Model of Therapeutics. *Journal of Loss and Trauma, 14,* 240–255.

Perry, B. D., & Dobson, C. (2013). Application of the Neurosequential Model of Therapeutics (NMT) in maltreated children. In J. Ford & C. Courtois (Eds.), *Treating complex traumatic stress disorders in children and adolescents* (pp. 249–260). New York: Guilford Press.

Perry, B. D., & Hambrick, E. (2008). The neurosequential model of therapeutics. *Reclaiming Childhood and Youth, 17*(3), 38–43.

Perry, B. D., & Pollard, R. (1998). Homeostasis, stress, trauma, and adaptation: A neurodevelopmental view of childhood trauma. *Child and Adolescent Psychiatric Clinics of North America, 7,* 33–51.

Perry, B. D., Pollard, R., Blakely, T., Baker, W., & Vigilante, D. (1995). Childhood trauma, the neurobiology of adaptation and the "use-dependent" development of the brain: How states become traits. *Infant Mental Health Journal, 16*(4), 20.

Pfeifer, J. H., Iacoboni, M., Mazziotta, J. C., & Dapretto, M. (2008). Mirroring others' emotions relates to empathy and interpersonal competence in children. *NeuroImage, 39,* 2076–2085.

Piaget, J. (1962). *Play, dreams, and imitation in childhood.* New York: Norton.

Ponkanen, L. M., & Hietanen, J. K. (2012). Eye contact with neutral and smiling faces: Effects on autonomic responses and frontal EEG asymmetry. *Frontiers in Human Neuroscience, 6,* 122.

Rizzolatti, R. (2005). The mirror neuron system and it function in humans. *Anatomy and Embryology, 210,* 419–421.

Schilbach, L., Eickhoff, S. B., Mojzisch, A., & Vogeley, K. (2008). What's in a smile?: Neural correlates of facial embodiment during social interaction. *Social Neuroscience, 3*(1), 37–50.

Shirk, S. R., & Karver, M. S. (2011). Alliance in child and adolescent psychotherapy. In J. C. Norcross (Ed.), *Psychotherapy and relationships that work: Evidence-based responsiveness* (2nd ed., pp. 20–91). New York: Oxford University Press.

Slobin, D. I. (1982). The role of play in childhood: In G. L. Landreth (Ed.), *Play therapy: Dynamics of the process of counseling children* (pp. 5–18). Springfield, IL: Charles C Thomas.

Szalavitz, M., & Perry, B. D. (2010). *Born for love: Why empathy is essential and endangered.* New York: Harper Collins.

Unger, M., & Perry, B. D. (2012). Trauma and resilience. In R. Alaggia & C. Vine (Eds.), *Cruel but not unusual: Violence in Canadian families* (pp. 119–146). Waterloo, Ontario, Canada: Wilfrid Laurier University Press.

van der Kolk, B. (2004). Psychobiology of posttraumatic stress disorder. In J. Panksepp (Ed.), *Textbook of biological psychiatry* (pp. 319–344). New York: Wiley.

van der Kolk, B. (2006). Clinical implications of neuroscience research in PTSD. *Annals of New York Academy of Sciences, 1071,* 277–293.

van der Kolk, B. A., Spinazzola, J., Baustein, M. E., Hooper, J. W., Hopper, E. K., Korn, D. L., et al. (2007). A randomized clinical trial of eye movement (EMDR), fluoxetine, and pill placebo in the treatment of post-traumatic stress disorder: Treatment effects and long term maintenance. *Journal of Clinical Psychiatry, 68*(1), 37–46.

Watts-English, T., Fortson, B. L., Gibler, N., Hooper, S., & De Bellis, M. D. (2006). The psychobiology of maltreatment in childhood. *Journal of Social Issues, 62*(4), 717–736.

Zigler, E. F., Singer, D. G., & Bishop-Josef, S. J. (2004). *Children's play: The roots of reading.* Washington, DC: Zero to Three Press.

Part II

MASTER CLINICIAN APPROACHES

The Sound of Silence in Play Therapy

Anne L. Stewart
Lennis G. Echterling

Silence in play therapy is a complex dynamic that can be particularly intimidating for beginning therapists, who may interpret this client behavior as an indication of their own ineffectiveness or as an expression of the child's defensiveness or hostility. Of course, responding therapeutically to silence can be challenging for experienced and new play therapists alike. Freud (1926/1978) popularized the term "talk therapy" and focused on the verbal communication in the relationship between therapist and client as the true essence of therapy, declaring, "Nothing takes place between them except that they talk to each other" (p. 6).

Play therapists, however, recognize the limits of language. In fact, play therapists treasure the transcendent possibilities of the wordless narratives that children can create through play. Yes, communication through language is an important therapeutic tool, but it often fails to capture adequately the deep, wired-in, and complex lived experience of the client. Children silently and eloquently communicate in a wide variety of ways—gesturing, frowning, smiling, grimacing, miming, crying, drawing, sculpting, using puppets, using sandtrays, writing, and playing are but a few of the countless ways—but whatever form their wordless expressions take, the process helps children to create meaning, add nuance, enrich, embolden, and personalize the therapeutic encounter.

In this chapter, we explore the possible underlying meanings of "clamming up" and discuss concepts that shed light on this common phenomenon of silence in play therapy. We describe a specific framework that we have found to be helpful in our interventions and place them in the context of case study examples. Finally, we share some concluding reflections on the potential for silence to be a rich and wordless expression that can provide a resonating, common healing space for a troubled client and empathic play therapist.

GENERAL APPROACH

Our general approach to viewing silence relies heavily on attachment theory, and also is influenced by a number of other perspectives, including anthropology, developmental psychology, and trauma-informed play therapy.

Attachment Theory

Attachment theory proposes that children's "attachment behavior system" leads them to seek proximity to their caregivers in times of physical or psychological distress, whether mild or severe, momentary, or long standing. In turn, caregivers serve as a safe haven of protection and as a secure base for children to use as they explore the world. The attachment system thus serves a biological function in humans, as in other species, of ensuring protection in dangerous surroundings, and also promoting exploration and learning (Bowlby, 1969, 1982).

From a practical point of view, as well as an evolutionary one, the immediate outcome of this pattern is that the child's physical and psychological needs are responsively attended to in the moment-to-moment emotional and behavioral episodes of the day. The more distal outcome, now evidenced through findings from neuroscience, is that the child's brain builds an increasingly sophisticated structure of neural connections. Satisfying interpersonal exchanges and corresponding dense synaptic growth produces comforting rhythms of soothing, co-regulation of thoughts, emotion, and behavior, and, over time, abilities for self-control and social competence. Children emerge from these interactions believing that they are known, seen, and valued; that adults are trustworthy and helpful; and that the world is exciting and safe to explore (Schore, 2001, 2005; Sroufe, 2005).

It is likely that you have realized a significant finding in both your personal life and in your professional career—attachment patterns are built one interaction at a time, over time. This is good news for children, caregivers, and play therapists. It appears both from research (Dozier, 2005) and from our clinical practice that caregivers with secure patterns, while not meeting all the child's needs all of the time, are able, through their own accurate perceptions and attunement to children's emotional signals, to help children form healthy attachment relationships through everyday interactions. Such caregivers, including parents, neighbors, teachers, mentors, and play therapists, provide an emotional environment that is sensitive, flexible, adaptive, responsive, and generally able to meet a particular child's unique needs.

Children with insecure patterns of attachment display poorly developed capacities for co-regulation (i.e., the ability to use caregivers for regulating their emotions and behaviors), ineffective mechanisms for soothing and self-control, and poor partnership behavior (Whelan & Stewart, 2015). In this regard, and through no fault of their own, children with insecure attachment patterns provide fewer clear cues about their emotional and relationship needs and caregivers experience children's behavior and feelings as puzzling and unpredictable. In these circumstances between individuals with unmet attachment needs, there is a high likelihood that silence, particularly in emotionally charged situations, will be hard to read or misunderstood by the caregiver or the child.

Anthropology

Anthropological studies have noted that silence is a socially constructed interpersonal phenomenon (Campo & Turbay, 2015). For example, many Eastern societies cultivate a more nuanced appreciation for silence in interpersonal encounters. Individuals in these cultures are more likely to tolerate, and even savor, such quiet times with others.

Moreover, the meaning of silence changes dramatically, depending on the circumstances and the relationship of those involved in the encounter. Silence may communicate respect to an authority figure, or it may indicate a comfortable sense of unspoken trust. On the other hand, silence may express defiance to a command that is perceived as unjust, or attempt to avoid emotionally painful material, or portray a profound sense of inadequacy to give voice to overwhelming emotions.

When successful, silence can actually give powerful expression to affect and also profoundly affect the relationship by creating a shared mind state. Thus it is crucial to consider cultural influences and the specific relational context in our child and family interactions. Contemplating what meaning silence may hold in a particular interaction during a session is an essential first step for the play therapist.

Developmental Psychology

Considering the child's stage of development is another important metric to consider. Does the silence reflect a developmentally appropriate reticence that is actually adaptive and not pathological? Is it signaling a need to actively push away, close down, or turn inward to gain emotional safety? The silence of a 3-year-old preschooler is likely communicating a dramatically different meaning from that of a 14-year-old adolescent. We encourage you to view "clamming up" as communication at any age.

Silence can also be an artifact or characteristic associated with particular developmental delays or diagnoses, such as autism, intellectual disability, auditory processing problems, hearing loss or sensory integration, and severe language disorders. The child may not be able to reliably process information received or consistently produce an appropriate verbal response. Comprehensive medical and psychological assessments and in-depth developmental histories can help rule out possible physical or sensory causes, examine cultural issues, and discover whether particular experiences or factors, such as learning English as a second language or a family history of anxiety, might be influencing the child's ability to respond verbally.

When silence is the referring issue to play therapy, we should investigate the applicability of a diagnosis of selective mutism (SM), a complex anxiety disorder characterized by a child's inability to speak and communicate in a developmentally and socially appropriate manner in particular social settings, such as school. For parents and teachers, a perplexing and often frustrating feature of SM is that the children do speak and communicate in settings where they feel safe, secure, and relaxed, such as at home. Common contributing factors for SM are anxiety and sensory processing challenges (Shipon-Blum, 2016).

The play therapy room can provide children many ways to maintain a tolerable level of anxiety and modulate their relational and environmental sensory exposures. A first step in lowering the child's anxiety can be accomplished by inviting both the child and a trusted person into the room (e.g., parent, sibling, or classmate). Accepting and responding to nonverbal communicative attempts, such as pointing, nodding, using communication boards, as well as replying to vocalizations and information from a "whisper buddy" or "supportive translator" can also reduce anxiety about using words. Incorporating strategies to develop the children's social communication skills will likely be necessary (Shipon-Blum, 2016). Frequent interprofessional consultation, along with supportive conversations with the family members and other concerned adults, can help lower pressure experienced by the child and increase the effectiveness of interventions across settings.

Trauma-Informed Practice

Most psychodynamically oriented therapists have interpreted silence as a client's resistance to forbidden emotions or to deepening transference. However, Ritter (2014) recently characterized silence as the voice of previous traumas and proposed that this disruption in communication may be a promising gateway to a client's traumatic experiences. In particular, such a silence may reflect the overpowering sense of shame that the client is reexperiencing in the session. Successful play therapy, therefore, can reverse the deadening impact of traumas by supporting the child in the sometimes frightening and painful process of healing. Un-silencing a child's threatening emotions through expressive techniques can promote the potential for resilience and recovery.

Attachment theory provides a useful conceptual foundation for trauma-informed practice. Infants are born with certain "wired-in" neuroaffective social needs that provide the scaffolding for attachments. Later, as toddlers and beyond, the realization that they are open to the negative judgment of others can aggravate feelings of shame. Throughout the lifespan, shaming experiences, such as ridicule or bullying, serve to continue feelings of humiliation. In fact, shame is the dominant emotion in interpersonal trauma (La Bash & Papa, 2014), such as sexual assault and child abuse. Posttraumatic stress disorder (PTSD) is typically characterized as involving irrational responses to external dangers. However, the perceived internal dangers—feelings of inferiority, worthlessness, inadequacy, and powerlessness—often lead to silence in therapy. The source of threat for a child who has survived a trauma may not be external. Rather, the child's silence can be a protective mechanism to ward off the interior threat of these unacceptable feelings.

As play therapists, we value how a person's entire body is an instrument of communication. Adolescents who engage in self-cutting typically find it difficult to adequately express their emotions in words and the silent, focused action of cutting uses the body as an instrument of communication (Straker, 2006). Unaccompanied by words, one's eyes, facial expressions, posture, and actions can articulate lived experience with both clarity and power. For example, a silence accompanied by unrelenting eye contact, pursed lips, aggressive posture, clenched fists, and jutting jaw portrays a defiant, oppositional stance. In contrast, a silence highlighted by a faraway gaze, wince of pain, sudden intake of breath, and frozen posture may depict a startle reaction to an intrusive traumatic memory.

Reactions to threats are often characterized as freeze, fight, or flight (LeDoux, 2015). In fact, silence may accompany any of these three self-protective responses to traumatic events. Trauma can leave one speechless. Collective silencing, in which society may blame the victim of a trauma or levy far-reaching institutional oppression, is another important possible dynamic to consider. In these and countless other situations, we are challenged to resonate empathically to such complex and endless variations on the theme of silence.

In summary, we find the framework of attachment theory, accompanied by concepts from anthropology, child development, and trauma-informed practice, provide a strong rationale for nonverbal-based interventions, such as the expressive techniques involved in play therapy. From an attachment-based perspective, silence may be seen as an adaptive and protective stance for children—a way to experiment with creating psychological space when an intervention feels intrusive. Equally, children might invoke silence to invite the therapist's help to co-regulate overwhelming emotions, bear witness to their pain, or punctuate a meaningful nonverbal narrative. Play therapy honors a child's development by providing a safe way to explore, express, and connect with the therapist. Using symbols and silence in play therapy, children can convey their disinclination to engage. Mandated, irate, shamed, or wary teenagers can effectively communicate their resentment, anger, humiliation, and reluctance through silence. Trauma-informed play therapy practices acknowledge that chaotic, physiologically encoded experiences may be safely accessed and processed with sensory interventions into nonverbal, play-based trauma narratives, rather than linear verbal trauma narratives.

Using music as a metaphor offers insight into the power of silence and its communicative intent in relationships. In music, a rest is an interval of silence between notes. Silence shapes and contours sounds, at times in order to echo the previous musical notes, and at other times to anticipate the notes that follow. Melodies are made of both sounds and silences that provide rhythm and cadence of the tunes. Composers use silence as a framing tool to accentuate and highlight the emotions that music can evoke. From an attachment theory perspective, the comforting gazes and sounds of cooing constitute a first language, establishing the connecting links between caregivers and infants. Describing therapeutic encounters across the lifespan, Amini and her colleagues (1996) relied on the music metaphor to observe, "The therapist has been invited to play in an affective-relational duet in which the patient's attachment patterns will provide the principal melody" (p. 234).

SPECIFIC TECHNIQUES

Communication is constantly verbal and nonverbal, cognitive and emotional, enabling play therapists to listen to clients using ears and eyes, head and heart. We actively dialogue with the child with words, and through gestures, vocalizations, facial expressions, and certainly by acknowledging and responding to the child's needs in play. Play is a creative and improvisational experience that generates feelings of well-being and trust, helping the therapist resonate accurately with the child's emotions and together create a therapeutic relationship. We believe this dynamic relationship is where and how the child and therapist compose their distinctive restorative and heartfelt melody of healing and growth, a LUV song.

Offer LUV

LUV refers to the LUV triangle, a graphic illustrating the fundamental principles for building any therapeutic relationship—those of communicating that you are listening, understanding, and validating (Echterling, Presbury, & Mckee, 2005). Play therapy practices can come across as gimmicks to a client if they are not offered with LUV (Figure 4.1). For this chapter, we intentionally redefined the listening apex to incorporate all the ways the child may be communicating with you, including "listening" to their silence.

We are extending the LUV theme to create a framework for our recommendations to remember to <u>h</u>onor, <u>e</u>xpress, <u>a</u>cknowledge, <u>r</u>esonate,

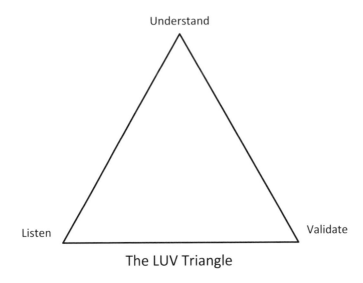

The LUV Triangle

FIGURE 4.1. The LUV triangle.

and track—HEART. The use of the HEART framework in play therapy is not meant to be prescriptive. We encourage you to apply it as a guide in recognizing and understanding children's needs in their unique context. HEART practice approaches can remind us to work with loving kindness and hope, to give HEART to each child.

Give HEART

Honor

Honor refers to recognizing the child's personal characteristics and relevant cultural dynamics of silence, recognizing its many possible meanings, acknowledging the limits of language. On a school playground in Costa Rica, I (ALS) noticed a young boy, about 6 years old, tucked in a small brick opening in the wall. He had developmental delays, and his slight frame just fit the spot in the wall. I admired how the hole provided a safe and secure place from which he could observe his classmates and me. He had claimed his own place of prospect and refuge (Dosen & Ostwald, 2013). Prospect and refuge theory describes how certain environments meet basic human psychological needs—in this case, a place from which to observe while feeling safe and protected. I was acutely aware of how much of an "other" I was to him—I was white, non-Spanish speaking, and a stranger. He was Costa Rican, and while he did not speak, he understood Spanish. I noticed he was moving some pebbles around on the ground so I sat down and, over time, also began to slowly move a small pile of pebbles in synchrony; I paused when he paused, I played with rocks when he played with rocks. I noticed he was watching with a faint smile, so I picked up a pebble, showed it to him, and then gave it a deliberate tap on the brick wall beside me. His smile grew wider. I looked at him and tapped the rock again. Lowering my arm, I looked at his pile of pebbles. He looked at me, smiled even more widely, grasped a rock and tapped it on the wall where I had tapped. This was followed by a big laugh. We engaged in variations of this conversation for more than 20 minutes, changing the intensity of the tap, the number of taps, and even exploring which pebbles could leave a mark on the bricks. No words had been exchanged, but a lot of communication had occurred.

Express

Express refers to scaffolding the child's communication and providing tools for sharing and exploring his/her emotional world. Playing, drawing, painting, sandtray, and other expressive therapies bring texture and richness to the therapeutic encounter. At times, silence may signal transderivational searches (Erickson, Rossi, & Rossi, 1976)—those mindful, introspective pauses during which children may tilt their heads and defocus their eyes as they explore their inner experience. During such silences, the play therapist may invite the child to engage in expressive play to access these unconscious processes.

Art is a powerful tool for providing silent children with the means to express themselves, especially if they are trauma survivors. Of course, multiple HEART practices can be present in an intervention, and in this instance the practice of honoring is crucial. Simply put, the therapist bears witness to the trauma depicted in the art and empathically reflects the possible feelings expressed in the picture. Before ending the session, the play therapist can also create opportunities for the client to give wordless expression to positive emotions, such as hope, determination, gratitude, and courage. You can say, for example, "I notice that this boy is helping to clean up after the fire. Can you draw another picture of how you helped?" Such questions invite children to become more aware of the depth and richness of their own resilience.

Accept

When we lead with acceptance, we validate children's experience and receive who they are with a welcome mat decorated with the word UNCONDITIONAL. Acceptance permits children to feel what they feel, think what they think, and act how they act, not in a free-for-all, but by sharing who they are in relationship with you. Your relationship assures them that they are not alone on their journey, that you will act in helpful and therapeutic ways to protect them from external and internal threats, and that you want to deeply know their emotional world.

A colleague was conducting individual therapy in the schools with Jamal, a 6-year-old Syrian boy. Jamal had arrived 3 weeks prior from a refugee camp and knew just a handful of English words. Not surprisingly, in class he vacillated between appearing curious and interested to downcast and despondent. Jamal's tentative exploration of the playroom was short lived. He soon found his preferred toys on the top shelf of a bookcase. His selection was an unlikely one in this well-stocked playroom. Jamal had spied a stack of five bath towels, not your typical playroom equipment. (The towels were stored in the playroom and used when the class went swimming.) Jamal methodically examined each towel and in an instant was on the floor. He placed the towels in a circle around him. Then, with great animation, he began to whip the towels around his head and body. Over the next 10 minutes, with varying intensity, Jamal rolled, hopped, and romped excitedly as he threw and retrieved the towels. The therapist demonstrated his acceptance of this unexpected activity with admiring facial expressions and supportive exclamations as Jamal continued to move around the room.

After the session, the therapist reflected on Jamal's play. While playing with the towels, Jamal's affect appeared to be primarily one of overexcitement, with no of evidence anger or distress. Could this behavior be related to trauma? Was it some form of stimulation? A hallucination? Classroom observations and information from the family did not indicate any neurological deficit or evidence of a thought disorder. While there were traumatic events in Jamal's history, he subsequently used playroom materials in ways that seemed relatable to the hurt he had experienced. For the next 7 weeks, Jamal played with cars, the doctor's kit, action figures, cooperative board games, and puppets in ways consistent with his lived experiences. And each visit to the playroom continued to include approximately 10 minutes of eager and purposeful (and mysterious to the therapist) play with the towels.

Words were beginning to be used sparingly in the playroom. Jamal was learning English faster than the therapist was learning Arabic, permitting the therapist to offer brief tracking comments. To Jamal's amazement, the therapist exclaimed, "عظيم", or "Wonderful" when Jamal proudly completed an operation on a puppet. By the eighth play therapy session, the therapist had located a qualified interpreter to accompany Jamal to the playroom. A transformation was about to occur with the therapist. As Jamal commenced his play with the towels, the interpreter translated his periodic shouts. The therapist quickly realized that each towel represented a specific character who possessed certain powers. Jamal was battling mighty forces and no winner was yet apparent. It appears that in the meager refugee housing, Jamal had created a world of play with the materials available (rags) and was continuing the combat in his new home. His imagination, inventiveness, and resilience were remarkable, and his need to battle superpowers made perfect sense.

Resonate

Communication that is tuned into the resonating wavelength between the client and play therapist is predominantly implicit, nonlinear, and without words. By responding to nonverbal overtures, play therapists accept an invitation to engage with the child in play that calls for emotional co-regulation—creating a deeply interpersonal experience. Behaviorally, you may be echoing sounds, drumming, mimicking expressions, or mirroring movements, while internally navigating an affective and somatic experience that expresses unquestionable empathy.

A compelling example of resonating with the child is illustrated in the high-stakes roller-coaster emotional experience of hide-and-seek. When informed that we had 5 minutes left in the playroom, Rosie, a 7-year-old girl referred for noncompliance at home and controlling interactions with classmates at school, abruptly stopped her dramatic play and asked if we could play hide-and-seek.

My reply, "It sounds like you know just what you want to do!", affirmed her choice. Rosie had been placed with a loving family for the past 5 years following an early start with parents with many stressors and little knowledge or energy to meet her needs. In an interesting and telling variation, Rosie's game of hide-and-seek involved her directing me, wordlessly and with some urgency, to hide her and then beckon her foster mother to enter the playroom and find her.

Rosie maintained control of the timing of her discovery by shaking her head no or tersely stating, "Not yet," if she was found too soon. At just the right time, signaled clearly by Rosie, this sensitive foster mother, who knew to voice what she was doing and seeing, would notice a chair out of place or the toe of a familiar-looking shoe to excitedly recover and embrace Rosie. They both expressed great delight and joy at their reunion, never adding any commentary on how Rosie orchestrated the event. The therapeutic value of this game of being lost and discovered, now under Rosie's direction, is captured by Marks-Tarlow's (2015) observation that "peek-a-boo and hide-and-seek both lurk at regulatory edges of abandonment fears. The danger of the Other potentially lost dissolves into the joy of the Other soon found" (p. 112). Truly resonating with a client in play therapy ultimately provides an unspoken reframing of children's worlds through their discovery of the Other in a safe haven.

Track

Tracking is a basic play therapy technique of describing the actions of the child engaging in play (Landreth, 2002). In the purest sense, tracking is acknowledging, paraphrasing, or describing whatever the person is doing. The technique is a fundamental part of the LUV triangle because following someone's emotional expressions, actions, gestures, or words can communicate that you are listening, understanding, and validating.

For many play therapists, the most challenging client they can contemplate is a silent teenager. We hope that, by this point in the book, you realize that even when not talking, the teen is communicating volumes. Now tracking can become your new BF (best friend). Similar to the stance adopted when watching a child play wordlessly in the dollhouse, you can wonder and comment on the many reasons the teenager is not ready to talk.

Depending on the affect presented you might offer:

"Seems like you're not ready to talk yet. My guess is that it wasn't your idea to come see me."
"Maybe you are not sure how to do therapy."
"You may be wondering whether you can just leave if you don't talk."
"Could be you are concerned I might ask you about things you don't want to talk about."
"You could be thinking that I'll tell your parents what you tell me."

And so on. This is another instance when returning often to LUV and offering many variations of the five HEART practices will be beneficial. Accepting the resentment or anxiety about being in therapy by clearly aligning with the teen in a therapeutic endeavor is crucial.

By tracking, you put your clients' silent communications into words, narrating their actions, gestures, and expressions. At a deeper level, you also are voicing empathically the unspoken strengths and coping skills that clients are demonstrating in play therapy. Well-timed tracking statements acknowledge the client's decision making and creativity in the session itself, which not only encourages the child to speak, but also promotes therapeutic momentum. Such here-and-now reflections are opportunities for children to see themselves in different, more positive ways. Body language, tone of voice, and facial expressions are often outside of the client's awareness. Therefore, the use of immediacy by tracking can reveal unexplored strengths and resources that provide the foundation for successful play therapy by building attachment and creating a therapeutic alliance. Ultimately, then, we can add one more "T" word to the practice of tracking—"T" for "treasure," valuing the transcendent possibilities of wordless narratives.

CASE EXAMPLE: TISHELLE—THE POWER OF WATER, THE POWER OF RESILIENCE

Nine-year-old Tishelle had not confessed this to anyone, not even her mother and father, but rooms without windows now gave her the creeps. When she first stepped into her new classroom after the hurricane, Tishelle quickly scanned it for a window. The classroom was a temporary one, a mobile home outfitted with desks, a blackboard, and an air conditioner that filled the only window. No escape was possible if floodwaters might come rushing through the door. Instead of a welcoming and safe classroom, it felt to Tishelle as oppressive and confining as a prison cell.

Before the hurricane, Tishelle had always been a quiet child and conscientious student. However, since the catastrophe, her new teacher noted with concern that Tishelle was nearly always mute, answering most questions with a nod or shake of the head—or, in rare instances, responding with a barely audible and minimal response. She was often distracted in class, gazing off in the distance, and vigilant to changes in the weather. Her parents have been worried that their once easygoing daughter now startles easily, becomes upset with separations, is obsessed with running water, and silently cowers whenever she encounters new situations. For these and many other reasons, both the teacher and the parents agreed that Tishelle could benefit from play therapy.

On the day that she would first meet her play therapist, Tishelle had been especially edgy. Nightmares often plagued her sleep, but this morning she was startled awake to notice that it was raining outside their temporary shelter. The raindrops seemed to strike the bedroom window with the ferocity of pellets that threatened to shatter the panes. To her deep shame, she noticed that she had once again wet the bed. Tishelle didn't mind changing and washing her sheets and pajamas. In fact, she hurriedly gathered them in the hopes that her parents might not notice this humiliating incident.

However, Tishelle's mother, who had become alert to the unmistakable sounds of her attempts to cover yet another bed wetting, gently comforted her tearful daughter with soothing words of "There, there, Baby. It's okay." Having led her to the bathtub, Tishelle's mother prepared her bath. Lately, it seemed to Tishelle that the water would gush out of the faucet with alarming force, growling with a malevolence that seemed almost gleeful in its rush to fill the tub with suffocating water. Tishelle stared with a mixture of fascination and dread as the bathwater rose higher to surround her legs. Although her mother tried to be gentle, washing Tishelle's face was especially disturbing. She jerked her head away, crying, "No, Mama!" whenever the washcloth brushed across her nose and mouth, momentarily blocking her breathing.

That afternoon, Tishelle discovered that the play therapy room was even worse than the classroom—it was both windowless and tiny. The oppressive sense of confinement stunned her when she entered the room with her mother to meet the play therapist. It was all she could do to remain there, taking long, slow, deep breathes to calm her nerves when her mother left her after introductions.

As the session began, Tishelle furtively cast her eyes about, silently estimating the distance to the door. She carefully scanned the play materials and made her way tentatively around the room, stopping briefly several times to pick up a toy and then carefully return it to its original position.

The play therapist sat on a small stool, leaned forward with her elbows on her knees, clasped her hands together, and gazed at the child with a calm smile. She shifted around on the stool to follow Tishelle as she slowly and silently circled the room.

THERAPIST: So, you're looking over some of the toys that are here in this room. [Tracking]

As the therapist speaks these words, Tishelle glances at her and returns to her exploration. Then Tishelle notices the sink in the corner and approaches it. As she reaches for one of the handles, she looks at the therapist with a questioning expression on her face, silently seeking permission to turn on the water.

THERAPIST: It looks like you want to be sure that it's okay to use anything in here during our time together. [Resonating]

Tishelle turns the handle, and jumps back from the splatter of the strong flow of water. She immediately turns it off and looks back to the therapist.

THERAPIST: Wow! The water splashed and you got out of the way! [Tracking]

Tishelle stands by the sink, gazing at the draining water, nodding and softly chuckling.

THERAPIST: It looked like it surprised you when the water came out so fast. [Accepting]

When the therapist notices that the child is managing her emotions, she joins Tishelle at the sink, turns on the water, steps back, watches the stream, and then turns off the faucet. [Resonating]

THERAPIST: Yep! That water can sure come out fast. [Honoring]

The therapist indicates that it is now Tishelle's turn to engage in what was becoming a ritual of repeatedly turning on and off the stream of water. She has improvised to use the sink as a tool for reenacting the child's experience. [Expressing]

THERAPIST: Now we're taking turns playing the water game. You turn the water on and off. And then I turn the water on and off. [Accepting]

The therapist narrates what has now become their collaborative play. As they continue taking turns, Tishelle becomes more controlled in her behavior so that the water stream no longer splashes out of the sink.

THERAPIST: Hey, Tishelle, you're learning just how to handle that water so it's not coming out too hard. [Tracking]

The therapist comments on the client's coping skills. After 10 more minutes of playing this interactive game, during which the therapist continues to offer HEART responses, Tishelle quietly sidles over to the table displaying paper and crayons.

THERAPIST: Yep, there's lots of stuff here for drawing. If you like, you can even draw yourself. [Expressing]

Without any specific directions or instructions from the therapist, Tishelle immerses herself in drawing a detailed picture of her family heading for shelter during the hurricane. She focuses on portraying the moment when she slips, but her parents cling tightly to her hands, and her father then lifts her above the threatening floodwaters.

THERAPIST: Oh my goodness! It looks like you, your Daddy, and Mama sure made it through a scary and dangerous situation. Tell me, what's going on in this part of the picture? [Resonating]

Tishelle pauses, looks into the therapist's eyes, and proceeds in a quiet voice to give a brief narrative. The therapist responds with LUVing curiosity and asks Tishelle to describe other parts of the picture, empathizing with the trauma narrative and being curious about the strengths she demonstrated in her survival story.

A few minutes before the session concluded, the therapist invited Tishelle to draw a picture of a happy memory that she wanted to keep. She drew a picture of her family together at the shelter with flocks of birds returning overhead to her community after the hurricane.

SILENCE IS GOLDEN

In this chapter, we have focused on a client's silence in play therapy. In our concluding comments, we wish to highlight the therapist's silence. One of the fundamental challenges for beginning play therapists is to appreciate the power of silence. The play therapist's quiet, resonating presence not only provides space for the child to engage in the healing work of play; it also creates a deep relational bond. A warm smile, tilt of the head, or a look of chagrin can all be silent communications of empathic engagement.

Instead of attempting to overcome the limits of language, the play therapist offers an eloquent, engaged silence that honors the child's immersion in the experience of therapeutic work. A quiet, even humble, presence gives the child space to engage in the creative process of making new neural connections and enhancing neuroplasticity. In contrast to the psychoanalyst striving to be a blank screen, the play therapist's silent moments are intended to communicate a deep, caring respect, rather than neutrality. In other words, silence is not merely a therapeutic technique. Rather, it is an honoring of the client's unique existence (Capretto, 2015).

One of the signs that play therapy is progressing well is when a client is silently resonating with the therapist. It is clear that the child is comfortable engaging in activities to which the play therapist bears wordless witness with empathy, warmth, and compassion. It is at these times that the silence is golden. There is no hint of "clamming up." Instead, there is a hushed encounter of awe and attunement.

FIVE RECOMMENDED PRACTICES

1. Honor—acknowledging the personal and cultural dynamics of silence, recognizing its many possible meanings, and acknowledging the limits of language.

2. Express—providing tools for sharing and exploring the child's emotional world. Playing, drawing, painting, sandtray, and other expressive therapies bring texture and richness to the therapeutic encounter.

3. Accept—validating children's experience assures them that they are not alone on their journey, that you will act in helpful and therapeutic ways to protect them from external and internal threats, and that you want to deeply know their emotional world.

4. Resonate—tuning into wavelength that is predominantly implicit, nonlinear, and wordless. By responding to nonverbal overtures, play therapists accept an invitation to engage with the child in play that calls for emotional co-regulation—creating a deeply interpersonal experience. You may be echoing sounds, drumming, mimicking expressions, or mirroring movements, while internally navigating

an affective and somatic experience that expresses unquestionable empathy.

5. Track—putting the child's silent communication into words by describing his or her actions, gestures, and expressions, expressing empathically the unspoken strengths and coping skills that the client is demonstrating in play therapy.

REFERENCES

Amini, F., Lewis, T., Lannon, R., Louis, A., Baumbacher, G., McGuinness, T., et al.. (1996). Affect, attachment, memory: Contributions toward psycho-biologic integration. *Psychiatry, 59*, 213–239.

Bowlby, J. (1969). *Attachment and loss: Vol. 1. Attachment.* New York: Basic Books.

Bowlby, J. (1982). Attachment and loss: Retrospect and prospect. *American Journal of Orthopsychiatry, 52*(4), 664–678.

Campo, A. R. R., & Turbay, S. (2015). The silence of the Kogi in front of tourists. *Annals of Tourism Research, 52*, 44–59.

Capretto, P. (2015). Empathy and silence in pastoral care for traumatic grief and loss. *Journal of Religious Health, 54*, 339–357.

Dosen, A., & Ostwald, M. (2013). Prospect and refuge theory: Constructing a critical definition for architecture and design. *International Journal of Design in Society, 6*, 9–24.

Dozier, M. (2005). Challenges of foster care. *Attachment and Human Development, 7*(1), 27–30.

Echterling, L. G., Presbury, J., & McKee, J. E. (2005). *Crisis intervention: Promoting resilience and resolution in troubled times.* Upper Saddle River, NJ: Merrill/Prentice Hall.

Erickson, M. H., Rossi, E. L., & Rossi, S. I. (1976). *Hypnotic realities.* New York: Wiley.

Freud, S. (1978). *The question of lay analysis* (J. Strachey, Trans.). New York: Norton. (Original work published 1926)

La Bash, H., & Papa, A. (2014). Shame and PTSD symptoms. *Psychological Trauma: Theory, Research, Practice, and Policy, 6*(2), 159–166.

Landreth, G. (2002). *Play therapy: The art of relationship* (2nd ed.). Muncie, IN: Accelerated Development.

LeDoux, J. (2015). *Anxious: Using the brain to understand and treat fear and anxiety.* New York: Viking.

Marks-Tarlow, T. (2015). From emergency to emergence: The deep structure of play in psychotherapy. *Psychoanalytic Dialogues, 25*(1), 108–123.

Ritter, M. (2014). Silence as the voice of trauma. *American Journal of Psychoanalysis, 74*, 176–294.

Schore, A. N. (2001). Effects of a secure attachment relationship on right brain development, affect regulation, and infant mental health. *Infant Mental Health Journal, 22*(1–2), 7–66.

Schore, A. N. (2005). Attachment, affect regulation and the developing right brain: Linking developmental neuroscience to pediatrics. *Pediatrics in Review, 26*, 206–211.

Shipon-Blum, E. (2016). Selective mutism and social communication anxiety. Retrieved from *www.selectivemutismcenter.org/aboutus/aboutus*.

Sroufe, L. A. (2005). Attachment and development: A prospective longitudinal study from birth to adulthood. *Attachment and Human Development, 7*(4), 349–367.

Straker, G. (2006). Signing with a scar: Understanding self-harm. *Psychoanalytic Dialogues, 161*, 93–112.

Whelan, W., & Stewart, A. L. (2015). Attachment security as a framework in play therapy. In D. Crenshaw & A. Stewart (Eds.), *Play therapy: A comprehensive guide to theory and practice* (pp. 114–128). New York: Guilford Press.

Play Therapy with Children Who Don't Want to Talk

"Sometimes We Talk, and Sometimes We Play"

Nancy Boyd Webb

Most children love to play and they do so alone, with peers, or even with adults. A trained play therapist knows how to use play as a means of communication, and although children usually talk when they play, language is not essential to carry out play therapy. A play therapist meeting a child for the first time typically states his or her name and then makes a statement such as, "I am a special kind of doctor (or person) who helps kids with their troubles and worries. Sometimes we talk, and sometimes we play. Your mother told me that you don't talk in school. You don't have to talk here unless you want to. You can look around the room and find something you want to play with and I'll just follow your lead."

The essential message of this introduction is to inform the child that the play therapist's job is to help the child, and that they will play together. The child is invited to select among a wide choice of toys and creative play activities; often, children are somewhat puzzled by this invitation to pick and choose, since it is far more common for adults to tell children what to do. The child may begin tentatively to explore the room and keep looking at the therapist to see if it is all right to take a doll from a shelf or to pick up a xylophone and start hitting the keys. Usually the therapist makes some reassuring general comments such as, "I see you are interested in the doll, or the xylophone," and/or, "Maybe you can find a bottle for the doll," or "Try playing some different notes on the xylophone." The point is that the therapist encourages the child to explore and play with whatever toys or activities he or she selects among the array in the typical playroom. As the child becomes more familiar with this situation, he or she gains confidence and eagerly explores the toy shelves and examines numerous toys before settling down to play with one or two items. Some children become very excited and stimulated when they realize that all the toys are available to them and they may have difficulty sticking with any one item. In situations like this, the therapist may comment, "There are a lot of choices and it is hard to decide, but you can pick something today and then try something different next time." The play therapist's stance is one of acceptance and encouragement.

The premise on which play therapy rests is that when the child understands that the therapist is someone who will help with his or her worries and problems while playing, the resulting play process will reveal the child's concerns. In other words, displacement and symbolism reside in the child's choice of toys, and the manner in which he or she uses them may reflect significant conflicts from his or her life.

This chapter focuses on play therapy with children who have been referred for help because they do not talk in school. The diagnosis of *selective mutism* (American Psychiatric Association, 2013) applies to such children who are nonverbal in specific situations, although they are capable of speaking and, in fact, may be appropriately conversant at home and in play with peers outside of school. Two cases will illustrate play therapy with children who were mute in school. In the first, the child's history included having a shy temperament and the possibility of sexual abuse in preschool; the second case involved the child's witnessing a traumatic event and the associated fears related to that. Both cases were treated with play therapy, which successfully resolved both children's mutism. The first case demonstrates the vital role of school and parental involvement in addition to individual play therapy sessions to help a mute child, and the second case combines play therapy with directive cognitive methods to create traumatic reenactments that resulted in crisis resolution and the resumption of the child's speech in the classroom. The chapter concludes with a summary of the treatment strategies that proved to be helpful in these two cases.

The incidence of selective mutism is very low (about 0.1%, according to the American Academy of Pediatrics; Kennedy, 2004), but many children remain undiagnosed because teachers tend to think that their lack of speech is temporary and due to shyness. Usually, the child's reluctance to speak becomes evident upon school entry, and the average age of diagnosis of selective mutism is between 3 and 8 years old. The condition may improve slowly for some children who appear to outgrow it. However, in serious cases the inhibition of speech with the accompanying stress and anxiety can lead to physical symptoms such as nausea or headaches, resulting in school avoidance and the child's subsequent social isolation. Treatments for selective mutism that bring symptom relief are discussed in the next section.

THERAPEUTIC APPROACHES

DSM-5 designates selective mutism as an anxiety disorder (American Psychiatric Association, 2013). Therefore, the goal of therapy is to reduce anxiety and build the child's self-confidence in order to facilitate his or her ability to communicate in social and academic settings. An individual treatment plan should be created that specifies recommendations about the role of the family and the school in collaboration with the child and the therapy process. Consensus strongly directs that the child *not* be pressured to speak by parents, teachers, or therapists, although the gradual resumption of speech is clearly the goal.

Individual factors in each case will determine the specific type of treatment for each child. The various choices include child-centered play therapy (Landreth, 2002), cognitive-behavioral therapy (Knell, 1993), crisis intervention play therapy (Webb, 2015), integrative play therapy (Gil, Konrath, Shaw, Goldin, & Byran, 2015), and medication. The cases described here demonstrate all of these methods, except the use of medication. Often, parents do not want to medicate their child and will do so only after other methods have not proven helpful. I have found that using a child-centered approach in the early sessions gives the child maximum control and comfort in relating to a strange adult. Later, after a supportive relationship has developed, other more directive methods can be implemented with the child such as positive reinforcement and gradual desensitization of anxiety through the use of audiotaping and relaxation exercises.

Often, children who do not speak in school also refrain from talking in therapy. This can present a challenge for the therapist, who must be able to tolerate the long periods of silence. The therapist knows that it will be counterproductive to put any pressure on the child to speak in the therapy sessions. However, when the therapist believes strongly in the possibilities of nonverbal communication through play, the therapy can proceed in its own unique manner. Many play activities, for example, involve pointing, or asking the child to nod "Yes" or "No," employing drawing, or movement, or music, without any use of words. It is also possible to play some board games, engage in sandplay, or make figures in clay or Play-Doh without any accompanying talk. Nonetheless, the therapist typically *does* talk and checks with the child to confirm whether his or her understanding of the child's meaning is accurate. There definitely *can be a range of nonverbal communications* between the therapist and the child, and over time, as the relationship develops the child usually becomes more trusting of the therapist and may permit, for example, the therapist to listen to a tape recording of his or her voice that was created at home. This activity, which requires the parent's participation, would not be suggested until the child was very comfortable with the therapist and the therapy process since it is essential for the child to feel that the playroom is a safe place and that the therapist genuinely wants to understand and help.

Parents and teachers often provide important collaboration in the therapeutic process. For example, in the case of Lisa, described below, the mother would record Lisa as she did her homework and then bring her to school early and meet for 15 minutes before class with the teacher in the hallway outside the classroom, where the teacher would listen to the tape in Lisa's presence. After Lisa became accustomed to permitting her teacher to hear her voice, she gradually began talking directly to the teacher. This case is discussed more fully below.

CASE EXAMPLES[1]

Case of Lisa

Family Information

Mother, Diana, 39, employed as a salesperson in a local boutique
Father, Albert, 40, employed as a stockbroker
Brother, Peter, 14, in middle school
Sister, Catherine, 8, in third grade
Client, Lisa, 5, in kindergarten
Nanny, Ursula, 55, speaks Russian and limited English

Lisa's parents emigrated from Russia when they were in their early 20s. All the children were born in the United States. This is a bilingual family who speak Russian with the nanny and English with one another.

---

[1]Names and certain details have been changed to protect confidentiality. Parents have given signed permission for me to write about the case for purpose of training professionals.

The Presenting Problem

Five-year-old Lisa was referred by the school social worker because she was not speaking in kindergarten. She spoke normally at home. The school was also concerned about Lisa's lack of peer contacts.

History of the Problem

According to the mother, Lisa began talking around 8 months of age and currently at home, she talks "nonstop." This is quite early, especially for a child who was raised with two languages. Mother began working when Lisa was about 2 months old, leaving the baby in the care of the nanny, who had been living with the family since Catherine's birth. The nanny was not fluent in English, so Lisa was exposed to two languages as she began talking. Children in bilingual families often have delayed speech, but they generally catch up. Obviously, this was not true in Lisa's case (Hamaguchi, 2010). Lisa was enrolled in nursery school when she was about 3½ years old and she didn't say anything there for several months. As time went on, she spoke very little, mainly saying "Hi" and "Bye." She changed schools the following year and she still didn't speak. The teacher referred the family to a child psychiatrist, who suggested medication, but the parents did not want to use medication, believing that Lisa was merely shy and that she would improve on her own. The following year in kindergarten, the school social worker suggested that the family consult a child therapist to deal with her mutism and they followed through with this suggestion.

Preliminary Assessment and Treatment Plan

After obtaining the family history from the mother as reported above, I saw Lisa for three individual sessions to formulate an evaluation. Lisa presented as a cute, lively child who did not speak, but who interacted enthusiastically with me. In the first session, she played eagerly with the dolls and the dollhouse and then initiated a game of tic-tac-toe, setting this up so that she won repeatedly. I experienced Lisa as somewhat controlling and oppositional. For example, after playing with the magic wand in my office, she put it in the pocket of her snowsuit jacket, intending to take it home; I stated that the toys stay in the office, and she reluctantly removed the wand from her jacket, looking annoyed.

In several sessions Lisa engaged the female dolls in hugging and kissing each other, but she would treat the male dolls harshly, often spanking them and throwing them on the floor. She remained silent during all of the early sessions, although she did communicate by shaking her head "yes" or "no" in response to my questions and a few times made some slight clucking/smacking sounds. When she reunited with her mother in the waiting room, Lisa would immediately whisper in her mother's ear.

It was clear that Lisa qualified for the diagnosis of selective mutism, which I conveyed to her parents with the recommendation that she participate in weekly play therapy sessions to try to help her feel less anxious about talking. The plan was for occasional sessions with the parents and the entire family in addition to individual therapy with Lisa. The therapist stated that she would confer regularly with the teacher about Lisa's school situation, and also indicated her plan to make a home visit in the future to meet the nanny.

Play Therapy Sessions

FIRST 3 MONTHS: APRIL–JUNE

Lisa was very engaged in therapy and seemed happy to participate. Her preferred activities were doll play, drawings, board games, playing with the magic wand, and making masks. She liked to hide and would often enter the office backward, holding her hands behind her and wanting me to guess what she had in her hands. Her play with male dolls continued to be very aggressive, and her drawings often depicted both male and female figures with their tongues stuck out; sometimes the male drawing revealed a penis exposed and hanging downward. Her hiding and secretive play, together with her aggression toward the males and open depiction of male genitals, made me suspicious about the possibility that Lisa had been sexually abused and told to "keep quiet" about it. Another possibility is that Lisa had age-appropriate interest in gender differences and that she probably had seen her teenage brother nude. It was impossible to verify either hypothesis, and I decided instead to focus on the presenting problem of mutism and to help Lisa become comfortable about talking in preparation for her entry into first grade the following September.

INVOLVEMENT WITH THE SCHOOL AND THE THERAPIST: SEPTEMBER–JUNE IN FIRST GRADE

Conferences with the school social worker and the first-grade teacher emphasized the importance of helping Lisa with temporary strategies to help her communicate nonverbally. In class, this included having cards on her desk indicating "yes" or "no" and a pass to go to the restroom. In addition, the teacher agreed to meet Lisa and her mother three times a week before school started and listen to a recording of Lisa doing her homework. This proved to be critically important in Lisa's development of a relationship with the teacher. After a few months, Lisa began whispering to her teacher and about halfway through first grade she began speaking to the teacher in her normal voice. She also gradually began speaking in class, although at first this was very limited and in a very low voice. Toward the end of the school year, the parents promised to take Lisa on a trip to Disneyland if she would read a story aloud to the entire class. She did this and was proud of herself. However, she continued to refrain from speaking to some boys at school, as well as to the school principal and librarian.

PLAY THERAPY SESSIONS DURING FIRST GRADE

Lisa continued to be very actively and eagerly involved in the weekly play therapy sessions. She remained mute while making drawings and playing the board games Candyland and Sorry!. She often laughed while she was playing, and reportedly had asked the nanny whether laughing is the same as talking. The parents were eager to bring the tape recorder to the play sessions so that I could hear her voice, and Lisa strongly resisted the first time her mother tried to play a recording of her voice in my presence. The mother insisted, and Lisa's defiance diminished in subsequent sessions when the mother continued to bring recordings. However, she still did not speak to me directly for several more months. Finally, she brought a book to a session and began reading it aloud in a very soft whisper.

My suspicions about possible sexual abuse resurfaced around this time, when she made two figures in Play-Doh, one a girl with a huge mouth and tears coming out of her eyes, and the other a male figure with a penis. She pierced both figures repeatedly with a toy knife and laughed and giggled as she did this. At the same time she clearly communicated pain and hurt with regard to the crying female figure. When I asked how we could make the girl feel better, she sketched the outline of a heart with a hole in the middle, which she attempted to look through. In a subsequent session after the family had gone on a ski vacation and I invited her to draw something about that, she drew two figures on skis, both with their tongues stuck out and one with a penis hanging out of his pants. Her affect during these drawings was quite animated and excited.

Tongues were repeatedly extended in most of her drawings, and when she spontaneously made a mask of a cat's face she cut out the mouth and then put it up to her own face and stuck her tongue out through the hole in the mask. She often drew two cats and sometimes would blacken out one cat, leaving the other intact. I wondered to myself if she had perhaps been asked whether "the cat had her tongue" and if she might have taken this expression literally.

SUMMARY OF PLAY THEMES

After several months of speaking to me in a soft whisper, Lisa came to a session in March dressed in her Halloween costume (a devil with a pitchfork) and used her normal speaking voice the entire session. She drew a picture of hearts and balloons with a sad face on one and then wrote a message saying, "I am not Lisa Romanoff" (her own last name; fictitious). I wrote back, "Then who are you??" She then wrote a different last name and moved to playing with a nude baby doll that she carefully dressed.

COMMENT

I was both very pleased and intrigued with Lisa's decision to finally communicate with me verbally, albeit as a devil in disguise. She seemed to be struggling with an identity problem; one could hypothesize that she felt partly bad (like a devil) and that she was trying to disengage herself from the "bad" Lisa by giving herself a different last name. I did not respond directly to Lisa's name change, but she may have experienced my lack of questioning as acceptance of her dual or different identities. In other words, although my own training and background led me to ponder the symbolism of Lisa's play, my overall stance with her was one of acceptance of the different facets of herself that she repeatedly revealed to me. She did, in fact, continue to create drawings with the two Lisas and referred to one of them (who was *not* her) as "a *bad* 18-year-old."

Summary and Concluding Comments

Therapy continued over the next academic year, with several vacation breaks. There was steady improvement in Lisa's participation in school, although she continued to avoid speaking to some male students and to selected school personnel. She was active in sports and piano after school, but did not have many friends. She clearly established a strong relationship with me and would write notes to me and/or make telephone calls during vacation breaks or when sessions had to be cancelled.

The treatment methods that helped Lisa included the various play therapy approaches that facilitated her communication, despite her inability to speak. Doll play and drawings were especially effective in encouraging the expression of good and bad feelings, which the therapist attempted to name and accept, leading Lisa eventually to be able to write some stories about these. In addition to the child-centered and some directed play therapy sessions, the therapist's consultation with the school created a collaborative focus for helping this child. Finally, inclusion of both parents in part of many sessions helped them carry through with the numerous tasks of supporting their child through her considerable anxiety-filled difficulties in overcoming her selective mutism. The case clearly demonstrates the power of play therapy as a vital communication tool with a nonverbal child.

There are definite challenges for the therapist in working with a mute child. The relationship seems at times to weigh heavily on the therapist's shoulders. For example, a therapist who knows that the child is verbal at home may come to resent the fact that he/she does not talk in play therapy sessions. At times, the therapist may wonder why the child does not trust him/her and may see the child as controlling and oppositional, as I did myself in the early sessions. However, when the therapist comes to realize that the child's symptoms are separate from the therapeutic relationship and rooted in deep anxiety, the task then becomes one of trying to understand the source of the anxiety and help the child move beyond it.

Lisa's play definitely presented her preoccupation with "bad" figures—either females or cats or males who were spanked and thrown on the floor. As I now review the details of this case more than a decade after treatment, I do believe that this child was probably sexually abused. In my more than 30 years as a play therapist only one other time did a female client repeatedly draw male genitalia, and in the other case the abuse had been confirmed. If I were treating Lisa now, I would ask her directly about the penises she drew and ask her to draw why they were out of the guy's pants. Whether the mutism was related to possible sexual abuse will never be known—but fortunately we do know that it was possible to successfully treat Lisa's lack of speech so that her education and social development could continue.

CASE OF SERGIO[2]

Family Information

Father, Manuel, mid-30s, heavy machinery operator
Mother, Nita, early 30s, cook and part-time babysitter
Client, Sergio, 9, fourth grade
Sister, Raquel, 3

---

[2]This case was published in detail in Webb (1999), with Teresa Bevin (1999) as the original author and therapist; it is presented in a shorter form here to illustrate how a traumatic/crisis event can precipitate the symptoms of selective mutism. Reprinted with permission from The Guilford Press.

The family was from Nicaragua. The father came alone to the United States to find employment and subsequently arranged for Nita and the children to cross the Rio Grande with a guide (a "coyote"), who was hired to assist them in their trip from Mexico across the border. The crossing proved to be difficult, and Nita slipped and fell and Sergio almost drowned. When they reached the other side, the coyote raped Nita at gunpoint while the children watched helplessly.

The Presenting Problem

Nine-year-old Sergio did not participate or speak in his bilingual classroom and he would not play with the other children in the playground. In school, he would become rigid and shake whenever the teacher tried to engage him. When the class went on a field trip, he refused to cross a small walking bridge over a stream and instead he sat on the ground and began to sob. Sergio's parents reported that he had bad dreams and often woke in the night and paced around the house.

Preliminary Assessment and Treatment Plan

Clearly, Sergio appeared to be responding to the multiple traumas associated with his immigration experience. The clinical team that evaluated him gave him the diagnosis of PTSD. The symptoms of selective mutism seemed to be related to his traumatic experiences. His mother had evidently told him to keep quiet about what happened or risk having the whole family deported.

    The treatment plan was for the therapist (a Spanish-speaking child development specialist) to see Sergio twice a week for play therapy sessions at school, and also to make home visits once a week to engage the parents as co-survivors of the trauma. The goal was to reduce Sergio's anxiety and panic-like reactions. The treatment methods would include various play therapy activities such as drawing, relaxation exercises, guided imagery, and journal writing, depending on Sergio's preference. The therapist believed that Sergio would need to engage in some form of traumatic reenactment after he had established rapport and trust in the therapist. The therapy was based on a combination of crisis intervention and cognitive-behavioral interventions.

Play Therapy Sessions

Although Sergio was mute in class, he did engage verbally with the therapist who had told him that her job was to help children with their worries and fears. The first four sessions were low-key, nondirected opportunities for Sergio to develop a sense of safety in the therapy process and to develop a relationship with the Spanish-speaking therapist who encouraged Sergio to play with whatever toys he wished. In the sixth session, the therapist brought out a plastic tub filled with water, a floating block, and some small toy figures. Sergio engaged actively in water play involving having a family of dolls swim and fish. In the following session, the same toys were laid out for him and the therapist directed a play scene in which the people have to go from one side of the tub to the other without the floating wood (boat). Sergio kept referring to the water as a swimming pool, but the therapist suggested that they think of the water as a river, and that the people had to cross it. He soon reenacted his own near-drowning experience, and during this play scenario he openly called for his mother, crying out that he was drowning.

In the following session, the therapist wanted to reenact his mother's rape, to which Sergio and his little sister had been helpless bystanders. The therapist facilitated this by bringing three rag dolls to the session (two males and one female); after Sergio played with the dolls for a while, the therapist asked the boy to show her what happened after he and his family crossed the river. At first Sergio resisted, but after the therapist emphasized his present safety, the boy reported that the coyote had a gun and that he pushed his mother to the ground and said some terrible things to her and attacked her. Later he took them to the safe house and his father came to get them the next day.

The therapist wanted to help Sergio release some of the negative emotions and fears associated with the traumatic event through several reenactment sessions. The therapist helped Sergio deal with his anger toward the coyote by encouraging him to attack the rag doll and tell him he should not hurt his mother. During this play, the therapist often repeated reassuring statements such as "You are safe now," and "It's all over now" to help the child put his haunting memories in the past. These reenactments definitely helped reduce Sergio's anxiety; his nightmares stopped and he began participating more fully in school. He continued in individual therapy for a year and later participated in group therapy with children who all were refugees.

SPECIFIC TECHNIQUES/INTERVENTIONS

These two cases illustrate very different underlying causes for the selective mutism of two children in their schools. In Sergio's case, the traumatic source of his mutism had been relatively recent, whereas Lisa had been mute in school for at least 2 years, since preschool. Play therapy was instrumental in helping both children, and although Sergio was able to talk in therapy, it is doubtful that he would have been able to reveal his traumatic experiences without the benefit of relevant toys and the gentle direction and reassurance of the play therapist.

In the case of Lisa, the therapist gave her free choice of toys she wanted to play with. This permissive, child-centered approach is particularly valuable when the therapist has no information about the possible source of the child's anxiety or symptoms. Although Lisa did not talk in therapy for the first year, she communicated definitively through her drawings and Play-Doh figures, as well as in playing with the various dolls. She clearly conveyed some of her conflicts and anxieties through this play, and although the therapist made no specific references to her own life, Lisa herself later in therapy drew pictures and wrote her name with a distinct suggestion about a past negative experience with an older girl with the same first name.

In addition to the play therapy sessions, the use of the tape recorder provided the opportunity to desensitize Lisa about permitting others to hear her voice. Initially, her mother's presence with the teacher outside of the classroom before school began offered a somewhat secure environment in which Lisa could sit on the sidelines and listen to her recorded voice in the teacher's presence. As she gradually became accustomed to having the teacher hear her speak, she was able to risk communicating directly with the teacher through whispering at first, and later with a soft voice. This process took several months and subsequently was repeated with the therapist. As already indicated, the cooperation of the parents and the teacher was critical in achieving Lisa's gradual ability to speak in school.

Sergio's case demonstrates the use of directed play therapy to encourage the child to reenact his traumatic experience. Similar to the protocol used in trauma-focused cognitive behavioral therapy (TF-CBT), Sergio's therapist provided toys that permitted him to recall and reenact his experience after being gently and repeatedly encouraged to do so. According to Neubauer, Deblinger, and Sieger (2015, p. 118), "TF-CBT has been proven efficacious in over a dozen randomized trials and has been cited in numerous reviews of the literature as having the strongest record of empirical support (Deblinger, Cohen, & Mannarino, 2012; Silverman et al., 2008)."

In retrospect, one might wonder whether it could have been possible for the therapist to direct some of Lisa's play with questions about why the tongues or penises were out. Of course, since Lisa was mute in therapy, any such queries would have had to ask her to draw another picture showing what the people were going to do with their tongues or penises. The fact that Lisa improved without any such delving into her own possible traumatic experience suggests that if indeed this had occurred, it was in the distant past and that Lisa felt safe in her present environment. Play therapy with selectively mute children involves a certain amount of speculation on the therapist's part, some of which may never be resolved.

At the time of this writing, an article appeared in the Science Times section of the *New York Times* (Saint Louis, 2015) about a group immersion program for children with selective mutism. Programs currently exist at Florida International University, Boston University, and at the Child Study Center at New York University's Langone Medical Center. All pair a mute child with an adult "buddy" with whom they spend 6-hour days, during which they participate in a variety of games and exercises in which the children are gradually required to answer questions and speak. The program refers to a "bravery ladder" in which each rung represents a step of increasing difficulty. Parents are involved at the beginning until the children become comfortable with the buddy therapists, and the programs last either over a weekend or for 6 days. The program reportedly is successful for many of the children, but not all. It definitely marks an awareness of the need to treat children with this unique diagnosis and it promises to lead to more awareness from the school and general public about the needs of selectively mute children.

In many instances, play therapy will continue to be the treatment of choice for selectively mute children. This book clearly demonstrates the validity of various play therapy methods to bring about considerable improvements in the lives of these anxious children who are afraid to speak and who are spending significant segments of their lives in silence. We hope that more treatment will be encouraged for these children in need.

FIVE RECOMMENDED PRACTICES

1. It's okay for the child not to talk. It's okay for the therapist to speak, but watch the child's face and body for clues as to whether he/she agrees with the therapist.

2. Trust the power of play for communication. Go slowly; don't rush.

3. Let the child take the lead with an activity. Don't push, prod, or try to cajole.

(continued)

FIVE RECOMMENDED PRACTICES (*continued*)

4. Have a range of toys available, including toy masks, hats of different types, and a variety of costumes. Some mute children will like to take on a pretend identity, and may speak through their pretend character. If this happens, it will be helpful for the therapist to respond to the child's fantasy persona, and not try to communicate with the child's true identity.

5. Trust the power of play for communication.

REFERENCES

American Psychiatric Association. (2013). *Diagnostic and statistical manual of mental disorders* (5th ed.). Washington, DC: Author.

Bevin, T. (1999). Multiple traumas of refugees—Near drowning and witnessing of maternal rape: Case of Sergio, age 9, and follow-up at age 16. In N. B. Webb (Ed.), *Play therapy with children in crisis: Individual, group, and family treatment* (2nd ed., pp. 164–182). New York: Guilford Press.

Cohen, J. A., Mannarino, J. P., & Deblinger, E. (Eds.). (2012). *Trauma-focused CBT for children and adolescents: Treatment applications*. New York: Guilford Press.

Deblinger, E., Cohen, J. A., & Mannarino, A. P. (2012). Introduction. In J. A. Cohen, J. P. Mannarino, & E. Deblinger (Eds.), *Trauma-focused CBT for children and adolescents: Treatment applications* (pp. 1–26). New York: Guilford Press.

Gil, E., Konrath, E., Shaw, J., Goldin, M., & Byran, H. M. (2015). An integrative approach to play therapy. In D. A. Crenshaw & A. L. Stewart (Eds.), *Play therapy: A comprehensive guide to theory and practice* (pp. 99–113). New York: Guilford Press.

Hamaguchi, P. (2010). *Childhood speech, language, and listening problems*. Hoboken, NJ: Wiley.

Kennedy, K. (2004). Suffering in silence. *AAP News, 24*(3), 126.

Knell, S. (1993). *Cognitive-behavioral play therapy*. Northvale, NJ: Jason Aronson.

Landreth, G. (2002). *Play therapy: The art of the relationship* (2nd ed.). New York: Routledge.

Neubauer, F., Deblinger, E., & Sieger, K. (2015). Trauma-focused cognitive-behavioral therapy for child sexual abuse and exposure to domestic violence. In N. B. Webb (Ed.), *Play therapy with children and adolescents in crisis* (4th ed., pp. 118–139). New York: Guilford Press.

Saint Louis, C. (2015, August 18). Scared into silence, little voices learn to speak. *The New York Times*, p. D1.

Silverman, W. K., Ortiz, C. D., Viswesvaran, C., Burns, B. J., Kolko, D. J., Putnam, F. W., et al. (2008). Evidence-based psychosocial treatment for children and adolescents exposed to traumatic events. *Journal of Child and Adolescent Psychology, 37*(1), 44–52.

Webb, N. B. (Ed.). (1999). *Play therapy with children in crisis* (2nd ed.). New York: Guilford Press.

Webb, N. B. (Ed.). (2015). *Play therapy with children and adolescents in crisis* (4th ed.). New York: Guilford Press.

6

Polyvagal–Informed Dance/Movement Therapy with Children Who Shut Down

Restoring Core Rhythmicity

Amber Elizabeth L. Gray
Stephen W. Porges

Psychic numbing may become a way of life, a debilitating character flaw. The person who lives his life in a place beyond expression, beyond feeling, will present a scary picture indeed. The absent eyes, the blunted responses to another response, these vacancies frighten anyone who recognizes what they really mean. Who lives behind the empty eyes? Sometimes— too many times—an ordinary child once lived there.
TERR (1990, p. 94)

Lenore Terr's groundbreaking work (1990) voiced an early understanding of the impact of terror on children. Articulated in behavioral terms, she describes the physical and emotional responses of a child who we can now describe as shut down or immobilized in fear from a polyvagal perspective. It appears that there are now more opportunities than ever for children to experience fear and terror and to live with imprints of overwhelming emotion. As clinicians, we may see these children in our practices as those who display flat or blunted affect; who do not speak and appear to be mute; who move with a frozen rigidity or lack of vitality that is ghostlike and sorrowful; or who clam up at the invitation to play or engage. These children may have encountered war or terrorism; long-term stays in refugee camps or fleeing dangerous situations; lack of access to educational resources and the basic needs of safety, protection, and nourishment; neglect and abuse by caregivers; or traumatic school violence.

Childhood is often looked back on as a magical time, but for some it is also a time of great uncertainty and exposure to threats and violence far beyond the child's ability to manage, cope, or respond. In a recent conversation with a supervisee at an early childhood, family, and community program where the majority of the cases suffer from some sort of interpersonal trauma exposure, the woman said, "I've been doing this work for 10 years, but have never read so many cases where the children have been exposed to horrors beyond my ability to cope, at such a young age." If this is the trend, psychotherapists, educators, and parents charged with protecting our children will need new and innovative psychotherapeutic practices that effectively restore safety, balance, connection, and hope.

This chapter explores the interface of the polyvagal theory with dance/movement therapy (DMT), a psychotherapeutic approach that is uniquely positioned at the crossroads of somatic psychotherapy and creative arts therapies. Following a brief overview, we present case material that illustrates a framework for polyvagal-informed DMT with children, which can be incorporated into clinical practice.

OVERVIEW OF POLYVAGAL-INFORMED DMT

Dance/Movement Therapy

DMT is a holistic approach to psychotherapy that integrates all aspects of the developing self: physical, emotional, cognitive, spiritual, and behavioral. It is also communal, social, and familial. To be alive is to be embodied, and to move is to explore the most basic language of humanity, the language we all begin with: movement. If movement is a primary language, then dance is the creative expression of our first language.

"Based on the empirically supported premise that the body, mind and spirit are interconnected, the American Dance Therapy Association defines dance/movement therapy as the psychotherapeutic use of movement to further the emotional, cognitive, physical and social integration of the individual" (American Dance Therapy Association, 2015). DMT has long recognized the potency of the nonverbal aspects of human development as fundamental to our becoming adult and becoming human in a fully integrated way. Maslow's (1943) hierarchy of needs is a useful concept to understand the somatic basis of development that DMT is uniquely positioned to address: With physiological and basic needs as the base of the triangle of our pathway to self-actualization, and safety as contingent on this physiological foundation, our journey to self-actualization begins and remains rooted in physiological processes.

DMT is a powerful therapy for working with children affected by trauma, especially those whose developmental trajectory appears to be disrupted. Development is functionally a creative process in which successful transitions reflect the integration of spontaneous exploration with a supportive social structure. This is where polyvagal theory and DMT converge; one need only observe the soothing and regulating interaction between a loving caregiver and a distressed infant to witness the neurologically and affectively regulating social structure provided by caregivers in a safe environment. These interactions that cultivate structure and containment are enhanced by periods of curiosity and exploration that guide a child's earliest movements. We begin our embodied lives in the horizontal dimension, lying on a floor, in a crib, and/or being protectively swaddled. The earliest movement explorations, such as orienting our head and face toward sounds or movements, initiate our rocking, "face-making," and sounding with our caregivers mirroring and attuning responses; we then progress to scooting and crawling, until eventually, we stand and begin to walk. This sequential developmental movement process becomes the neurosequential, sensorimotor, somatically based foundation of our sensing, feeling, thinking, and action. These are the earliest underpinnings of our interoceptive and exteroceptive capacities. In fact, if we describe the developmental trajectory of childhood as an embodied, creative process, then the disruption of this process instigated by wounding, trauma, or disease can only be restored somatically and creatively.

The Polyvagal Theory

The polyvagal theory illuminates the role that the autonomic nervous system plays in guiding relationships between humans, and between humans and the environment (including all people present in the environment), by mediating safety through a process labeled neuroception (Porges, 2011). This theory, and its ongoing discoveries and contributions to clinical practice, elucidate that safety and human connection (and perhaps more broadly our capacity to love another) may be the most essential ingredients of a "successful" therapeutic relationship and process.

The polyvagal theory emphasizes how the evolution of the mammalian autonomic nervous system influences human behavior. It describes social engagement as an emergent, spontaneous, and adaptive behavior regulated by a specific neural circuit found only in mammals that developed though the evolution of the neural regulation of the autonomic nervous system in vertebrates. Similar to several other vertebrates, mammals have an autonomic nervous system with sympathetic and parasympathetic components. However, the vagus, a cranial nerve and the primary component of the parasympathetic nervous system, has two branches (dorsal vagus and ventral vagus, described later). These two branches plus the sympathetic nervous system provide three autonomic circuits that support three broad classes of behaviors: social engagement, mobilization, and immobilization.

The polyvagal theory is based on an understanding of the behaviors and functions that emerge from the three autonomic circuits or pathways described above. The two branches of the vagus nerve are the dorsal vagus (i.e., the phylogenetically "old" vagus) and the ventral vagus (i.e., the phylogenetically "new" or "mammalian" vagus). Both branches provide motor fibers that exit the brainstem together packed inside the vagus nerve. The vagus is a large cranial nerve that serves as a conduit conveying neural fibers that enable bidirectional communication between the brain and virtually all of our visceral organs. In addition to these two motor vagal pathways, the vagus contains an abundance of sensory fibers informing the brain of the status of the visceral organs. Within the vagus, the primary motor pathways of the dorsal vagus travel to the organs below the diaphragm and the primary motor pathways of the ventral vagus travel to organs above the diaphragm. Thus the dorsal vagal branch is often known as the subdiaphragmatic vagus and the ventral vagal branch is often known as the supradiaphragmatic vagus.

The primary target organs of the ventral vagus are the heart and bronchi, which enhance oxygenation of the blood and promote states of calmness. The primary target organs of the dorsal vagus involve the organs of digestion and reproduction. A primary function of the dorsal vagus is to support homeostasis and to regulate digestion. Note the use of the term *primary* in the above sentences, since both branches send fibers above and below the diaphragm. To help clarify this potential confusion, the vagal motor fibers originating in brainstem source nucleus of the dorsal vagus (i.e., dorsal motor nucleus of the vagus) are not myelinated, while those originating in the brainstem source nucleus of the ventral vagus (i.e., nucleus ambiguous) are myelinated. This structural difference has important behavioral and adaptive consequences. Myelin is a coating on the nerve that enables it to convey information more rapidly. For example, the dorsal vagal pathway is involved in regulating massive decreases in heart rate and blood pressure in response to life threat.

These physiological responses enable the cessation of behavior and an inanimate appearance.

The polyvagal theory also offers new insights into the relationship between attachment and safety, especially in early childhood, as the foundation that enables us to live a life informed by meaningful relationships and the positive social engagements that promote well-being during childhood. An understanding of the clinical, restorative, and healing implications of the polyvagal theory are essential to any psychotherapist working with children affected by trauma, especially those who clam up and shut down.

The Social Engagement System

The social engagement system describes the physiological and biological dynamic neurological processes that underpin and guide our interactions with the environment via the vagus nerve. The social nervous system refers specifically to the five special efferent (motor) pathways that regulate striated muscles (somatomotor). These cranial nerves (V, VII, IX, X, XI) innervate striated muscles arising from the bronchial arches (descendants of primitive gill arches) and provide the neurophysiological mechanisms for facial expressivity, prosody of voice, posture, affect, and gaze. These "signs of engagement" are key areas of intervention that DMT is uniquely poised to support, as illustrated by the casework presented in this chapter. Also relevant to DMT, the area of the brainstem in which the ventral vagus emerges is involved in the regulation of the striated muscles of the face and head. This creates an integrated social engagement system that includes anatomical structures for vocalizations, facial expression, listening, and ingestion. In other words, these are the structures that "move" our face in service of nourishment, human connection, and expression. In the brainstem, the neural regulation of these structures is linked to the vagal regulation of the heart. Vagal regulation of the heart through the ventral vagus functions as a "brake" to slow heart rate. For most of us, due to the tonic influence of the "vagal brake" on the heart, our heart rate is usually much slower than the intrinsic rate of our heart's pacemaker. Effective functioning of the vagal brake is linked to the expressive potential of DMT interventions to promote social engagement through face-to-face contact and communication.

John Hughlings Jackson (1882) described dissolution (evolution in reverse) as a basic principle of the nervous system's response to injury and disease. Polyvagal theory incorporates the Jacksonian principle of dissolution to describe a similar phylogenetically ordered hierarchy in how the autonomic nervous system reacts to challenges. The autonomic nervous system responds initially with ventral vagus and the social engagement system as a mode of social communication. This circuit uses facial expressions, vocalizations, and gestures to communicate and maintain calmness in a safe context and forms a basis of human relationship. When the social engagement system is not recruited, the body is prepared for defense. Under these conditions, there is removal of the vagal brake and a simultaneous dampening of the entire social engagement system, which causes the upper face to become affectively flat and reduces intonation or prosody of voice. This change in state promotes hypervigilance for danger and provides the neurobiological conditions for fight–flight to be initiated through activation of the sympathetic nervous system.

The two branches of the vagus, including the sensory information traveling from our organs to our brain, have profound effects on the regulation of autonomic state as a neurophysiological platform for safe or threatening situations. For safe social interactions, defensiveness is reduced by increasing the prohomeostatic functions of the ventral vagus. In contrast, in dangerous and life threatening situations, the ventral vagal influence is withdrawn to potentiate the expression of either the fight–flight (via sympathetic nervous system) or immobilization (via dorsal vagal pathways) defenses when we face danger or life threat. In many situations, such as during physical restraint when there is no option to escape, fight–flight strategies are not effective. In these situations, an ancient defense system may reflexively shut us down. This strategy involves the dorsal vagus, which reduces our metabolic demands and raises our pain thresholds to reduce suffering in the face of perceived life threat. Immobilization with fear may be manifested as fainting or as states of dissociation.

Finally, the heart and brain are efficiently connected through the ventral vagal pathway that regulates the heart and bronchi via myelinated motor fibers and receives sensory information from the face, head, and heart that is sent back to the brain. In addition, sensory information evaluating the status of visceral organs below the diaphragm is traveling through the dorsal vagus. This dynamic bidirectional communication influences how we think, feel, and behave as the brainstem interprets information from our body and informs higher brain structures.

The Gut–Brain Connection

The gut–brain connection, via the dorsal vagus nerve, is of special importance to somatic and creative arts-based psychotherapies. Body awareness (i.e., our ability to sense our "inner landscape" and our "place in space and time"), informs us what is going on inside our body and how our body relates to gravity, objects, and others in the environment. For clinicians working with traumatized children, our clinical intuition, which draws from this "inner knowing," is an essential guide to how we track, respond, and engage with our young clients, who, either due to their developmental timeline (i.e., how old they are) or imprints left on them by traumatic exposure, may be unable to describe their inner world, or may be disconnected from their ability to sense and feel their own bodies. Many trauma survivors describe the body as both a mine-field and a place of refuge, and the tendency of traumatic exposure and the fear response that can "lock the body down" in a physiologically based fear state, makes access to a safe refuge challenging and some-times seemingly impossible. A strength of working somatically is an abil-ity to promote the shifts in physiological state that are instrumental in shifting emotional and psychological state. Simply stated, it is impossible to shift the way we think, feel, or perceive the world if we don't shift physiological state.

The state shifts that are central to this theory depend on the three autonomic circuits described above: ventral vagus, sympathetic nervous system, dorsal vagus. This process of dissolution, during which social engagement is compromised in the service of survival, occurs when we face danger and mobilize in fight–flight or face life threat and immobi-lize. In the moment of response, these adaptive strategies, which often save our lives, are provided by our evolutionary lineage and operate out-side our day-to-day awareness.

Neuroception

Neuroception (Porges, 2004) is an essential process that enables the body to rapidly shift autonomic state to match environmental challenges. It is part of an ancient survival system that detects risk outside the realm of awareness. Basically, we need not be conscious of the cues of risk that trigger shifts in biobehavioral states that optimize our survival in safe, dangerous, and life threatening contexts. The word *neuroception* differs from perception, which implies a conscious awareness of the cues, and differs from sensation, which emphasizes the features and not interpre-tation of the stimulus. Basically, neuroception triggers implicit processes in our brain, below the layers of language and explicit awareness, that cue us to whether we are safe or not. Neuroception helps organize our feelings, intentions, and underlying physiological state to move in and out of environments and relationships, to deal with risk, and to optimize our ability to feel safe and connected with others.

During the entire lifespan, feeling safe is an antecedent to trust and is fundamental to the establishment of meaningful and reciprocal

human relationships. The vagal pathways play a central role in our sensing safety in the space we move through (environment), the people we
share the space with, and how objects and people make us feel. Children
rely on primary caregivers early in life for this sense of safety; developmentally, we co-regulate with another before we self-regulate. Children
affected by trauma, especially those who are shut down, have lost their
ability not only to self-regulate, but also to co-regulate with those around
them, especially if primary caregivers were involved in disrupting their
sense of feeling safe. This lack of self- and co-regulation manifests in
a dysfunctional social engagement system, which influences behavior,
movement, and intentionality of action.

Relationship and the Social Engagement System

The social engagement system can simply be described as the structures
enabling us to convey our own physiological state to others. The acoustic features of our voice and our facial expressiveness signal our physiological state to others. For example, a high-pitched vocalization signals
distress, anger, or fear. When we hear someone else shriek or yell, we
may feel unsafe, especially if that person is someone we trust to keep us
safe. When we experience fear and terror our facial expressivity changes
and our faces becomes less expressive. We have a "flatter" or less dimensional expression when we are afraid, especially when we shut down and
dissociate. When we witness this lack of expression in others, we may
become concerned as well, and our ability to connect and engage may
degrade.

Our social engagement system enables us to be calmed by the
soothing voice of another and to actively attempt to self-soothe by eat-
ing and drinking. Looking into a "safe face" can also provide comfort.
Especially relevant when working with children, expressive faces can
amuse, engage, and promote playfulness. Since the brainstem regulation
of both the muscles of the face and the ventral vagus define the motor
pathways of the social engagement system, we can track in real time
the dynamic shifts in physiological state, trust, and openness by observing facial expression and listening to our clients' voices. These features
(i.e., facial expressivity and vocal intonation) of reciprocally interacting
social engagement systems are particularly employed in successful interpersonal relationships, including effective therapeutic interaction, with
strong social connectedness.

Social engagement refers to a core element of our ability to experience meaningful, supportive, loving relationships. It enables opportunities of shared feelings and a common intersubjective experience. As
humans, the social engagement system enables relationships to develop

as we start our journey as newborns. This process of building relationships through active and reciprocal social engagement behaviors continues throughout the lifespan and is an important defining feature of being human. While the selective relationships with primary caregivers figure predominantly early in life, the same interactive reciprocal processes involving the social engagement system are involved throughout the lifespan. The products of these interactions provide the primary source of feedback from which we continue to develop, grow, and create meaning. Metaphorically, the explicit outer world defined by the success and failure of our social engagement and inner worlds experienced by the implicit shifts in physiological state that occur during social engagement interactions are always dancing together in service of our individual development and species evolution.

THE FRAMEWORK FOR POLYVAGAL DMT

On April 20, 1999, as I (AEG) was preparing to share my "Shadow Project," inspired by my time working in post genocide Rwanda, with my very soon-to-be-graduated class in DMT, news of the Columbine School shootings broke. Days later, my then-supervisor asked if I would be able to work in Leawood Elementary, the school next door to Columbine, because the social workers assigned to assist the schoolchildren process what they had experienced were challenged by the children's apparent unwillingness to speak. The social workers thought some "nonverbal therapy" might be helpful.

Brand new and right out of graduate school, I showed up at Leawood 8 days after the shooting, armed with puppets, stretch bands, bouncing balls, and art materials. I didn't know where to begin. The dance/movement therapist has, as her most powerful "tool," herself. Our movement, our sensation, our somatic awareness is our internal guide; our strongly developmental theoretical framework is our foundation. In each classroom, and in sessions with smaller groups of children or individuals whom the school social worker flagged as in distress, and even in the lunchroom, I sat with children and listened, and then offered toys, puppets, and drawing materials to help them begin symbolizing what they were feeling. This was the segue to movement. While movement is truly our primary language, no matter what our cultural heritage is or what language we eventually speak, the symbolic realm is the intermediary language between movement and spoken word. It is often more "relatively safe" (A. St. Just, personal communication, 1998) to begin with the symbolic realm when working with young survivors of trauma, especially those who clam up and don't speak. The internal intimacy of the sensate world can be too provocative if explored too early in treatment. Whether due to age and development, or the non- and preverbal nature of traumatic experience and memory that is now well documented (Herman, 1997; Porges, 2011; Rothschild, 2000; Siegel, 2012; Terr, 1990; van der Kolk, 1994; van der Kolk, Hopper, & Osterman, 2001; van der Kolk, 2014), for many children who shut down timing of somatic methods and approaches is crucial to the client's ability to tolerate physical sensation and feeling states that are deeply rooted in the body. Beginning with the symbolic realm, therapies that support safety and stability are the hallmark of the "best practice" phasic approaches to treatment for complex trauma especially those occurring in childhood (Herman, 1997; van der Kolk et al., 2001).

The most challenging classroom was the one with the youngest students (kindergarten). They were frozen. The teacher had asked to speak with me in advance, and told me the level of fear in her classroom "stressed her out" to the point of feeling overwhelmed and helpless. She didn't know what to do. The kids were afraid to go out to the playground, because a policeman was patrolling with a gun on his hip (later, the policeman and I held the ends of the school's very long jump rope so all the kids could jump rope and experience him as "safe person," there to protect them). She asked me to speak with the children. So I began with general questions about what they were learning in school; questions about some of their art hanging in the classroom; and I talked about knowing they had been through a very scary time and wondered how they were feeling. They spoke very little; their faces were frozen in wide-eyed fear.

I invited them to draw, and so we scribbled for a while; a few of them began to draw red and dark colors, and images, so we talked about "bad people who shoot people" for a while. This is when the fear the police officer was causing them emerged. Everything froze again.

At this point, early in my career as a dance/movement therapist, I was not familiar with the polyvagal theory. So I stood there for a moment, lost, and then based on clinical intuition and my need to move beyond stuckness, I decided that it was time for us all to move. I was aware of a charged energy moving inside of me, and yet I was standing there, very still, like the energy in the room. It was uncomfortable. *I needed to move.* In retrospect, I would refine what I did in that moment based on what I now know from this theory. But here's what I did, and here's what happened:

"Hey kids, do you like this classroom?"

"Yes!"

"Okay; do you feel safer here, or outside?"

"Here."

"Great; you ever play games in this classroom?"
"YES!"
"Does it feel safe enough to play games in here today?"
Pause. "A little bit."
"Okay. What would make it safer?"
Another pause, and then one of the children said, "A HUG."

I was surprised, and not sure what to do. So I asked, "Who do you want to hug?", at which point the entire room screamed the teachers name, and ran to her, in a massive small-child-hug-pile-on.

The energy in the room had shifted. Based on what I now know, it had shifted from immobilization in fear to mobilization in excitement, which was much more tolerable as we could begin to dissipate the fear that permeated the classroom. They had to move to hug the teacher, and the movement resulted in giggles, contact, play, and more movement. We began to play "push me–pull you" games after the group hug (see Table 6.1). We were playing, and in the energy of play, we were reconnecting, socially engaged, initiated by a collective hug.

The state shifts that occurred in that moment are the core of poly-vagal-informed DMT. In order to shift emotional and psychological states, and for those state shifts to manifest as therapeutic change, it's necessary first to shift physiological state, and movement is a key to shifting physiological state. If you move, your autonomic state recruits sympathetic excitation, and when in a state of sympathetic excitation, the dorsal vagal pathways are inhibited and you *cannot* shutdown. Moreover, if you use face-to-face interactions while mobilizing, the social engagement system will constrain the mobilization and link it to play and not fight–flight behaviors. As dance/movement therapists, we have multiple skills, methods approaches that enable and promote these state shifts.

THE DMT BRIDGE TO THE POLYVAGAL THEORY

Embodied Presence

This section covers DMT skills and strategies that bridge clinical work with the polyvagal theory. These strategies include embodied presence, breath, movement repertoire and affective expression, kinesthetic empathy, state shifting, the developmental progression, and core rhythmicity. One of our skills is embodied therapeutic presence. In the words of Geller and Porges (2014),

> The Polyvagal Theory proposes that a state of safety is mediated by neu-roception, a neural process that may occur without awareness, which

TABLE 6.1. Push Me–Pull You: Yield, Push, and Reach

The push me–pull you activity is based on the basic neurological actions and developmental progression described on page 121.

Yield

Ask the children to find a partner (preferably someone close to their own size to begin; this can change) and stand side by side. Invite the children to rest and settle, or ground, or grow roots into the earth. so that they are in an "relaxed alert" posture.

Invite the children to lean into each other, shoulder and side body to shoulder/side body. Then cue the children to yield into one another:

1. "Feel your feet connected to the floor [earth]. Grow strong roots into the floor, so you can stand strong."
2. "Lean into each other so that you can feel the support of your partner. See how much you can relax into your partner while still 'standing strong.' "

Processing questions: "What does it feel like to have someone to lean into?"; "How long do you think you could stay here?"

Push

Children remain in the same dyad; while they are settling more into their yield, enthusiastically "shout":

1. "Now PUSH! Push as hard as hard as you can into your partner! Push! Push! Push! Notice what happens to the support you felt when you pushed. Notice if you are about to push your partner over or be pushed over."
2. Take a break.
3. Switch partners and do the same sequence (settle/ground, yield, push). Invite the children to experience yield but suggest that one partner "collapse" while pushing or being pushed; and that one partner "stiffen" while pushing or being pushed.

Processing questions: "How did pushing against your partner feel different than leaning into your partner?"; "Did you notice a difference between the collapsed push, the stiff or rigid push, and the supported (yield) push?"; "What did you do with your body to avoid being pushed over?"; "Which strategy was more effective [yield, collapse, or stiffen]?"

After the group has completed this with two to four partner switches, we shift to reach, grasp, and pull.

Reach, Grasp, and Pull

1. "Face your partner and stand arm's length away."
2. "Reach your arms out and grasp your partner's hands. Make sure you have room to really extend your arms out in a reach action."
3. "Reach your arms long, and while holding [grasping] hands [or wrists] kneel down as low as you can go, without letting go of your partner. If you fall or break hand contact, start again. See if you can sense when you might pull on your partner while reaching and moving up and down."
4. "Once you have done this in a pair, try it in fours, then groups of 8, 12, 16 and more. . . ."

Process questions: "Do you feel any yield or push when you move like this, while reaching toward your partner?"; "Could you sense the difference between reach and pull?"; "Were there times you pulled?"; "What made it possible to do this with bigger groups?"

constantly evaluates risk and triggers adaptive physiological responses that respond to features of safety, danger, or life threat. According to the theory, when safety is communicated via expressed markers of social engagement (e.g., facial expressions, gestures, and prosodic vocalizations), defensiveness is down regulated. Cultivating presence and engaging in present-centered relationships can therefore facilitate effective therapy by having both client and therapist enter a physiological state that supports feelings of safety, positive therapeutic relationships, and optimal conditions for growth and change. (p. 178)

The dialogue that resulted in the group hug (which I was later asked to join) began with my sensing, internally, the "collective" physiological state in the room. In polyvagal language, despite a colorful and cozy environment in the kindergarten classroom, the children's faces and body movements appeared afraid and shut down. They were uncharacteristically immobilized; the worry and fear imprinted on their faces reduced any sign of facial expressivity that is characteristic of playful engagement; they seemed hesitant to move, and moved in small "personal orbits" or "personal space bubbles." These personal space bubbles are what a dance/movement therapist refers to as a kinesphere, that is, the space in which we feel safe and comfortable to explore the environment around us. They can literally shrink for those who are traumatized, because we are neurocepting the features of danger, even when there may be safety in the space around us.

Breath

My response was to catch my breath, center and ground myself, and then slowly introduce energy into the space. From a polyvagal perspective, breathing is a portal to engage and exercise the regulation of the ventral vagus. When we slowly exhale, we are functionally activating the calming influence of the ventral vagal circuit, which functions as the "enabler" of our interactive social engagement system. Thus, the consequence this simple voluntary behavior of "catching my breath" resulted in my face and social communication becoming more animated. Every word was also spoken with gestures; I intentionally made faces to punctuate my words. And I sequentially made eye contact with every child and with the teacher. I also used my body to gesture and to move the words I was speaking, a practice I refer to as *body prosody*. Body prosody, by expanding and "innovating" one's movement repertoire, can support enlargement of a shrunken kinesphere. It can also shift physiological states from fear-based states to non-fear-based states.

Movement Repertoire and Affective Expression

Another core premise of DMT is that body movement reflects the inner emotional landscape (Kornblum & Halsten, 2006). Physical change like change in movement behavior, posture, and muscular tension will have an effect on emotional functioning. Unlike practitioners of traditional forms of psychotherapy, dance/movement therapists recognize and consciously reconnect the intricate and undeniable connection between people's history, thoughts, feelings, behaviors, and their bodies (Levy, 2005). These changes in movement behavior, posture, and muscular tension can now be understood as aspects of Polyvagal "Rules of Engagement" (Porges, 2013a), which include posture during social engagement, mood and affect, facial expressivity, gaze, and vocal prosody. As movement therapists, we are perhaps uniquely trained to observe and intervene at the level of movement or body prosody, which might also be described as movement repertoire. It is perhaps the prosody of our bodily expression, as shared through movement and dance that determines our repertoire and our nonverbal interactions with others. Using these basic principles of DMT, I was actually promoting state shifts in myself, and then inviting them for the children, from immobilization in fear to mobilization without fear; the latter is illustrated later in Figure 6.5.

Kinesthetic Empathy

Kinesthetic empathy, which was DMT pioneer Marian Chace's term to describe the nonverbal somatic expression of empathy between a client and therapist as demonstrated by mirroring and attuning, can be utilized to promote safety in the features or signs of social engagement: posture, sounds, facial expressivity, and prosody. In the practice of kinesthetic empathy, meeting and understanding the client in movement (Chaiklin, Lohn, & Sandel, 1993), the therapist becomes a mirror—witnessing, and reflecting the nonverbal expression of the client. Mirroring and attunement, which are essential components of healthy attachment and co-regulation between caregiver and child, are the basis for the development of a healthy nervous system with accurate neuroception of the features of safety in other people that enable the establishment of trusting relationship. These concepts are particularly useful in treating trauma survivors and serve as the basis for the ability of older children and adults to modulate their feeling states and regulate their emotions within their relationships. This convergence of social bonding with the process of co-regulation is embedded within the polyvagal theory as stated in the following quote:

To develop a social bond, individuals have to be in close proximity. This is true for the models focusing on both mother–infant attachment and the strong bonds associated with social monogamy. Both models test the strength and features of the relationship through separation paradigms." (Porges, 2011, p. 188)

State Shifting

Figure 6.1 illustrates the hierarchy of physiological states proposed in the Polyvagal theory. Physiological state moves through this hierarchy as neuroception detects environmental cues shifting from safety, to danger and life threat. As illustrated in Figure 6.2, changes in behavior parallel the immediate influence of neuroception on physiological state. The behavioral changes reflect adaptive shifts to match the environmental demands as they shift from the safe co-regulation with another, to mobilized fight–flight behaviors, and finally to a total behavioral shutdown in which the individual is protected from the predator by appearing to be inanimate. This hierarchical sequence may be presented as a "traffic light" image in which the safe ventral vagal state is represented as the top light, the mobilized fight–flight sympathetic nervous system state as the middle light, and the inanimate features of a dorsal vagal state as the bottom light. The traffic light image may be used in querying children about their internal physiological state, since children are familiar with the inherent meaning of these symbols and colors. The top "light," which represents the green light (instead of the usual red), or "go," reflects a state in which social engagement occurs spontaneously. This state involves the ventral vagus and the social engagement system. The second light from the top, which would be yellow in a traffic light, or "caution," reflects a state that is vigilant for danger cues and requires sympathetic–adrenal activation. The bottom light, which represents the red or "stop" light in this diagram, reflects a state of immobilization in which the child becomes inanimate in order to disappear and hide from a predator. This behavior is coordinated with the dorsal vagal pathway. Working with children, we often use a "safety thermometer," or this traffic light picture, and ask them if they feel free to move, play, and interact (green–go); afraid enough to run away or fight (yellow–caution); and so afraid they want to hide or run away (red–stop).

The state shifts promoted by the polyvagal informed DMT methods described here are illustrated in two formats. Figure 6.3 shows a simpler version that demonstrates the hierarchical dissolution that occurs when faced with danger or life threat, and the ensuing need for survival. The mammalian nervous system has evolved to promote social engagement

Polyvagal State

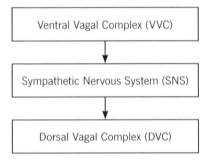

FIGURE 6.1. Hierarchical model of polyvagal states. Copyright © 2016 by Stephen W. Porges.

(green, or the top light) as a state of well-being, calm, and relationship in a safe environment. The ventral vagus complex (VVC), which is the most evolutionarily recent neural circuit or "branch" to develop in the nervous system's development, has an inhibitory or "braking" effect on the sympathetic nervous system, which promotes mobilization (fight–flight) as a behavioral strategy when we face danger. The "spinal" sympathetic system is first evident in the darting movement of bony fish. The term *spinal* is introduced to emphasize that the sympathetic nervous system includes ganglia that parallel the organization of the spinal cord and function in coordination with the spinal nerves regulating our skeletal muscles.

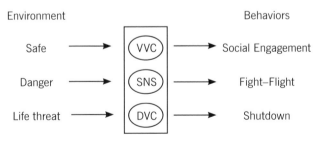

FIGURE 6.2. Neuroception: Matching physiological states with environmental cues. Copyright © 2016 by Stephen W. Porges.

The VVC's inhibitory action on the sympathetic nervous system allows us to maintain a state of social engagement in safe, soothing, nurturing environments. This "yellow" state (the middle light) is a state of readiness, defensiveness, and alertness in fear; it also describes a state of play when fear is absent (see Table 6.2). The bottom light, immobilization ("red") is the oldest behavioral strategy for survival that our evolutionary past affords us. This complete shutdown occurs when the old, or dorsal, vagus basically puts on the "brakes" to all systems that would require metabolic resources, resulting in a state of immobilization. In humans this is also experienced as dissociation, often without the biobehavioral shutdown that would lead to fainting or defecation. When we face life threat and experience terror, this is a fear-based immobilization that is our last chance for survival. In a non-fear-based state, when the dorsal vagal pathway is not recruited in defense, dorsal vagus can support homeostatic processes including deep rest, blissful surrender, or "rest and settle." As illustrated in Figure 6.4, when our neuroception detects safety, the sympathetic nervous system and the dorsal vagus are not recruited in defense, but can now support physiological homeostasis (e.g., health, growth, and restoration) and behaviors of play and intimacy.

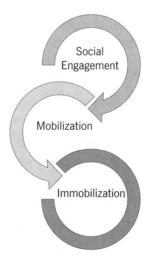

FIGURE 6.3. Dissolution as a hierarchical shift in adaptive biobehavioral states when faced with danger and life threat. Copyright © 2016 by Stephen W. Porges.

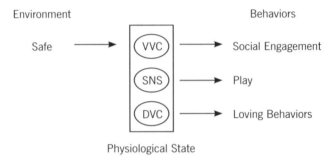

FIGURE 6.4. Neuroception: Safe environments expand the range of social behavior. Copyright © 2016 by Stephen W. Porges.

The words in Table 6.2 serve as a nonexhaustive example of various client and therapist descriptions of these states. The power of polyvagal-informed DMT is in the ability of the work to shift physiological states, from fear to non-fear-based, in a way that may simultaneously circumvent and honor the responses the body has adapted in service of survival. When children are shut down, they are immobilized in terror. All too often, well-meaning therapists can promote social engagement too quickly, thus triggering trauma memories and another fear response. While the dissolution that occurs at the biological level is truly in service

TABLE 6.2. Polyvagal States: Evolution in Action

	Risk/fear	Safety/no fear
Social engagement system	Depressed social engagement while orienting to threat: alert, cautious, heightened senses, increased tension and orientation	Feelings of mutual connection and reciprocity, engaged, ease, safety, relaxation, calmness, alert, present, curious, responsive, receptive
Mobilization	Hyperaroused, anxious, manic, angry, enraged, panicky	Playful, energized, laughing, excited, active
Immobilization	Unfocused, disconnected, depressed, dissociated, frozen, flat affect, shut down	Open, serene, calm, restful, mellow, able to cuddle

Note. Adapted from Harrison (2015) with permission from the author.

of our survival, the pathway back to healing and restoration may not follow the developmental trajectory. It is not as simple as backtracking along the evolutionary pathway; we may literally need to shift from a fear-based state to another fear- or "excitement"-based state (i.e., immobilization to a more competitive mobilization, with just enough excitement in place until defenses can be carefully deconstructed). Or the shift may go directly from mobilization in fear to mobilization without fear. There is not a one-size-fits-all formula, but DMT offers many options for shifting states through movement, rhythmic activities, kinesthetic empathy (Levy, 2005), sounding, and increasing movement repertoires (or vocal and body prosodic attunement) that talk therapy simply does not.

In Figure 6.5, the pyramid shows how three body states that are part of this polyvagal-informed DMT framework support social engagement. Many trauma-informed, evidence-based, and best-practice approaches include "somatic" methods, and most focus on "relaxation" or downregulation. Only recently, with the input of somatic psychology

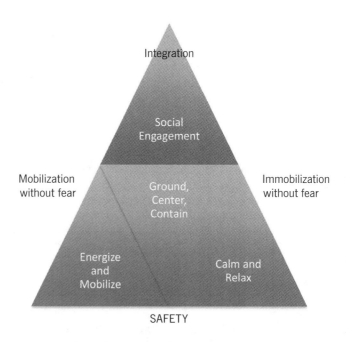

FIGURE 6.5. Fluidity and variability in up-, down-, and side-shifting of body states promotes modulation, regulation, balance, social engagement, well-being, and integration. Copyright © 2016 by Amber Elizabeth Gray.

and DMT, are the more mainstream approaches recognizing that both up- and down-shifting are essential to promoting physiological state shifts that increase safety and stability, and mastery over one's own body responses, enough to support the processing of traumatic memories and meaning making (Gray, 2015). The three states shown have many "substates"; however, in the work of DMT, they are three fundamental physiological states that are important to access whenever we need to shift our state in support of action or rest. The states are described here as ground and center, calm and relax, or energize and mobilize. Ground and center is a state of sensing one's connection to, and support from, the ground; it's a state that promotes connection to one's embodied core strength. Calm and relax may seem similar to ground and center; these are states that more closely approximate states of rest, settling, and eventually, sleep. DMT historically has referred to these types of states as energy states, and in the work of movement pioneer Bonnie Bainbridge Cohen (2012), the free and fluid movement of energy throughout the body is visible in the sequencing of energy visible in the developmental movements that all humans explore in the sensorimotoric journey from womb to mobile adult.

The Developmental Progression

Dance/movement therapists track the sequencing of energy through endpoints (places where energy enters and leaves the body): head (ventral vagus and the social engagement system), pelvic floor (subdiaphragmatic dorsal vagus), hands and feet (sympathetic nervous system to support mobilization). We observe and intervene with a development progression of movement (yield, push, reach, grasp, and pull) and the basic neurological actions (BNAs) that track our ontogenetic and phylogenetic development. It is beyond the scope of this chapter to present Bainbridge Cohen's work in depth, but her work highlights how human development is intricately linked to both our species evolution made visible in the earliest movement explorations of infants and toddlers; and that each individual's developmental trajectory contains the BNAs associated with fish, amphibian, reptile, and mammalian movements. The BNAs clearly link DMT assessment, diagnostic and intervention tools to the polyvagal theory. Each of these sequential movement phases contain the energetic or state memories of the experiences we encounter and encode in our early childhood.
    Variability and flexibility in an individual's ability to "call up" and fluidly embody states, such as relaxation or excitement, are movement-based determinants of well-being and social engagement. Our ability to

ground, center, and contain supports all energetic state shifts, whether we up, down, or even "side" regulate. Well-being and a state of social engagement might be described as accurately appraising the environment, through accurate neuroception, to appropriately move toward or away from features in the environment (which includes persons and situations). Our physiological state literally determines how we move through space. In states of well-being and engagement, we move fluidly and interactively. In states of fear, our movements will show either the fear of mobilization/fight–flight, or the terror of immobilization/shut down and clammed up (see Figure 6.6). From a developmental perspective, these states are linked to body memories encoded in our earliest years. The memory, or imprint, of experience allows us to access these states as body resources when we need them in response to current demands or features in the environment.

Early childhood trauma truncates the progression through the BNAs, the developmental sequencing of movement, and the full development of,

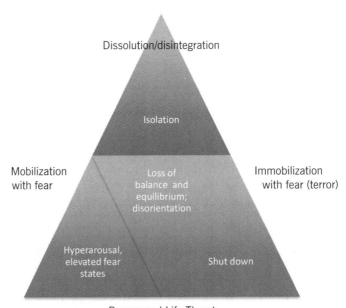

FIGURE 6.6. Loss of fluidity in up-, down-, and side-shifting of body states reduces and restricts modulation, regulation, balance, social engagement, well-being, and integration. Copyright © 2016 by Amber Elizabeth Gray.

access to, and expression of physiological and emotional states. Simply put, childhood trauma disconnects us from our ability to modulate our emotions and regulate our states in whatever environments, people, or situations we encounter and move through. Figure 6.6 illustrates how this loss of fluidity increases our risk for disintegration and isolation.

Core Rhythmicity

The core rhythms that underpin these states and promote well-being are heart rate (60–80 beats per minute), respiration (one breath every 3–5 seconds; 12–20 breaths per minute), and vascular feedback/rhythmicity (every 15–30 seconds). Oscillations of rhythms, especially when they are reinforced by externally changing tempos (as can be facilitated with the use of culturally congruent music) can provide a feedback loop to core rhythms of the human body. These rhythms all change in states of social engagement, mobilization (which can feel and appear like fast, sharp, or energetic movements), and immobilization, which can feel and appear slow or heavy, like molasses. Movement as felt experience and as it may appear to an observer, requires shifts in autonomic state that are manifested in changes in heart rate, heart rate variability, respiration, and vascular feedback to slow down or speed up and maintain fluidity.

Berrol (1992) summarizes several studies that demonstrate how rhythm affects physiological responses: "Emotional perception of music has a significant effect on autonomic responses—e.g., changes in pulse rate, galvanic skin response, and blood pressure. Bodily rhythms and activities appear to regulate to external rhythmic stimuli, matching tempi, which can help regulate emotions" (p. 25). From a polyvagal perspective, a slow exhale calms and slows down: "A slow exhale is the respiratory process associated with expressing special vocalizations" (Porges, 1995, 2007). This enhances VVC impact on the sinoatrial (SA) node, which is how the VVC enervates the heart and inhibits the SA and expresses the increase in cardiac vagal tone. A faster breath and shorter exhale enable the sympathetic nervous system to upregulate the heart and energize us. Because the primary influence on our core rhythmicity is our biology, the observations of therapists working in many cultures inform us that culture is a secondary but profound influence. As we develop, cultural experiences influence how we express emotions, move in and out space, what music we listen to, how we dance and posture, and tell us whether eye contact and facial expressivity are socially acceptable with strangers or in public. The indicators of social engagement (facial expressivity, gaze, prosody, mood/state, and posture) are the primary ways we communicate safety; facial expressivity, prosody, and gaze are literally reflections of our heart (Porges, 2007, 2009). It's not language, but rather our biology that communicates safety. Fear is the final layer that can undermine the biological and cultural influences on our core rhythmicity. These concepts and strategies are perhaps best illustrated in a case example.

CASE EXAMPLE: ALPHONSE—FROM SHUT DOWN AND CLAMMED UP TO SOCIALLY ENGAGED

Background and Clinical Presentation

Alphonse was a 13-year-old male from a region of West Africa long engaged in civil conflict. He had endured separation from his family of origin and his extended family in the last 6 years of his life, when war raged in his region.

Alphonse was reunited with his family in the United States, and they brought him to see me at a torture treatment program where I served as clinical director. When I met him, he was completely immobilized. He was mute and shut down, with no detectable kinesphere; he refused to look at me and refused to engage. His parents had managed to get him to school for a few days at a time, but he was so awkward and socially isolated kids made fun of him, so they pulled him out. When Alphonse was provoked he would flash into a rage state, hit someone, and then shut down again. There was no intermediary state for him. I truly had never been in the presence of a child whose behavior was almost animal-like in its unpredictability and lack of human features of safety and engagement. He exhibited deficits in vocal and body movement prosody, eye gaze, facial expressivity, lack of affect and affect modulation and regulation, and posture. His standing movement was sluggish and light at the same time; when he sat or lay down, he became heavy. He was so slumped and withdrawn, physically, that whether he was sitting or standing, he literally appeared to be disappearing.

I invited Alphonse to my therapy space, which in my opinion was a wonderfully safe place, full of color, musical instruments, toys, and plants; I assumed it was a safe space for all. My other child clients looked forward to their "playful therapy" with me. Not Alphonse. Every time he came to see me, he sat down in a chair, or lay on the floor, and collapsed. He refused to speak. I would put different props and objects out, play music, or try to engage him in movement or talk. Nothing.

After the fourth session like this, I spoke to his father when he arrived to pick him up, and informed him that I did not believe I could help. His father begged me, with tears in his eyes. He said, "You have no idea what this child has seen. It's as if the horror has eaten him. Please try."

I asked him if he noted anything that helped bring Alphonse out of his silence at home. He said that sometimes Alphonse would talk a little when he hid under a piece of furniture. That gave me an idea.

Safety and Environment

The next time Alphonse came for his appointment, we met in the front room of our offices, which were housed in an old Victorian structure. The front room served as a second waiting room, and was simply furnished: one large round table with four chairs, and a small bookshelf with a few books. It was sparse. At the time, it occurred to me that it would be a useful place to meet, as he could hide under the table. Later, I realized that the lack of stimulus, what might be called the "Zen" quality of the space, may have promoted a sense of relative safety for him far more than the excitement of my very colorful, vibrant therapy space. Given his immobilized physiological state and disconnected emotional and psychological state, this environment was probably a better match with his nervous system, and one that his neuroception would evaluate as relatively safe.

The move changed everything. Alphonse came in and immediately crawled under the table, collapsing on the floor. I found my beginning point—a collapse exists when there is an absence of yield, our first task in the human physiosomatic developmental sequence of movement (Bainbridge Cohen, 2012). Yield reflects our relationship to gravity, and gravity is a force that truly is always present. Yield supports us to relax and settle our weight into the earth; it also supports us to mobilize and push off the earth if we need to. Yield is an immobilization without fear state and action, and it precedes push in the developmental sequence; push is when we begin to use the grounding of yield to explore our weight in verticality and establish boundaries, which requires increased energy and mobilization. Push supports our ability to reach for what we want and retreat from what we don't want. When we reach for what we want, we can grasp and pull it toward us, literally and energetically (Bainbridge Cohen, 2012) in an act of social engagement.

The Social Nervous System and the Developmental Progression

I lay down next to the table and modeled a yield by "resting and settling." I played with resting on, and then pushing up, from the floor so Alphonse could see me. This small movement exploration engaged my spine in the BNA of spinal push and reach, much like early fish movements. At times, I exaggerated these so Alphonse could see the movements. It's possible that the flexion and extension of the spine in these actions promotes vagal tone, because sacral neutral has been shown to promote vagal tone (Cottingham, Porges, & Lyons, 1988).

Alphonse became interested in exploring movement with me for the next several sessions. As he imitated me resting, rocking, pushing off, and eventually "lizarding" through space, we also began to connect through our gaze more frequently. As this evolved naturally, I held his gaze initially for just a few moments, and then consciously increased the length of time I looked at his face. I began to make faces. As I began to make faces, he began to make noise. At first they were quiet animal like grunts and sniffle-snorts; over time, they became louder vocalizations, never quite a yell, but loud. Sometimes they were staccato and quick; other times they were sustained. I began to respond in increasingly more rhythmically varied vocalizations, and after four sessions, so did Alphonse. As I shifted rhythmicity to a more fluid vocal prosody, so did he, although this was challenging for him. A month later, we were communicating through a more fluid and prosodic sound and movement stream, with a few brief conversations occurring from time to time.

As we began to relate to one another through developmental movements, sound, and facial expressions, I introduced a physio-ball, which promotes pushing with yield versus pushing with effort. I placed it between our feet and pushed it, encouraging him to push against it as well. This homologous push of the feet is an early (reptilian) developmental movement that we repeated until it sequenced from feet to head, engaging the spine. We alternated between co-pushing the ball between our feet, and him pushing his head (spinal push from the head) into the ball, which was against a wall. We still spent most of our time together on the floor, but his movements were increasingly more coherent and fluid, and he traveled throughout the room, then retreated back to his hiding place under the table. I maintained a steady presence, tuning in to him and varying kinesthetic mirroring with kinesthetic attunement (responding in my own way vs. mirroring him exactly). I shifted from mirroring to attunement to restore this important somatic developmental task, and to promote an increase in his movement repertoire and kinesphere. After 12 weeks of weekly sessions, he frequented his hiding place a little less.

State Shifting and Engaging Language

I recognized that Alphonse was beginning to connect to me because smiles began to emerge on his face, and he held my gaze much longer.

There was increased vitality in his movements, which gradually shifted from always being floor bound and collapsed, to a blend of yield, push, and reach in more vertical postures. He showed state shifts, varying from his original immobilized in a nonresponsive, flat affect, to increasing his physical ability for strong push movements with increased energy that were accompanied by sounds that had an almost angry tone, often with a defiant face. When I mirrored or attuned to these sounds, I exaggerated my facial expressions and movement in accompaniment. Sometimes his movements appeared lighter and more playful and were accompanied by a smile. A few times, a wistful look appeared when he would pause in stillness and sit staring into space as if lost in thought.

Overall, he began to demonstrate more range in his kinesphere and more variability in his movements, movement rhythms, and emotional states.

When Alphonse did retreat to his hiding place, I would try to speak with him. We did not engage in long or complete conversations, but he began to answer questions such as:

"Alphonse, you look pretty comfortable under there."

"Yes."

"How do you feel right now?"

"Okay."

"Just okay?"

"Tired."

"How does your body know it's tired?"

"I'm heavy. I can't get up."

"Have you felt this way before?" And so on. It was through these sparse conversations that I began to gather a little information about his emotional world, and then was able to begin speaking to him about how he looked (i.e., collapsed or strong posture) and how he felt (sad or calm). He eventually remembered not being able to get up when he hid during a mass amputation in his home village; he described being so afraid he stopped feeling and didn't move for fear they would hurt him. We began to differentiate between when he felt like this in the past, and when he felt this way now. When he seemed to understand that his frozen experience saved him, we worked on strategies to remember that now it was usually safe for him to move. The strategies included pushing with strength and making a loud sound if he needed to; humming (soft or loud, depending on who was around), and kicking until he could push off the floor or a wall. He could also take a breath and scrunch his face up on the inhale, then he let it out slowly, making a face and sounding like a balloon. He often laughed when we did this; this is when "polyvagal balloon buddies" (described later) were born.

I believe these brief conversations helped Alphonse connect his body experience, or body narrative, to his affective states, which allowed us to connect a little more. They also helped him distinguish past from present. This weaving together of body narrative, affective states, and verbal communication contributes to the construction of a more integrated narrative. Listening to my own body cues to guide me into rest or movement invited Alphonse to vary his posture and activity, and eventually to experience more fluid transitions between rest and motion.

Core Rhythmicity

Three months into treatment, I asked Alphonse if I could play some music. My rationale was polyvagal, since listening to music is a trigger to the neural regulation of the middle ear muscles, which are enervated by cranial nerves V (trigeminal) and VII (facial). Middle ear muscles regulate a peripheral filter of sounds and influence our ability to detect sounds that signal safety or danger. Cranial nerves V and VII are both included in the five cranial nerves that comprise the social engagement system. Listening to music and the external tempo associated with music can restore internal rhythmicity (Berrol, 1992). He agreed. I played some music from West Africa; he didn't like it, so I invited him to bring some of his own music next week and asked his father to remind him.

Alphonse arrived with a favorite tape. When we began to play the music as a backdrop to our movement and sound dialogue, a shift occurred: he began to dance. At first he rocked on the floor; then he swayed and rocked in a seated position, while he hummed along with the music. Taking his cue, I sat, hummed and swayed with him, then I stood up and began to dance in slow, swaying movements. He joined me. We continued for 20 minutes, then he silently sat down again, looked at me, and took a deep "rest and settle" breath, and smiled. Something inside him had shifted.

This session birthed "polyvagal play stations." For the next 6 weeks, I began to set up these play stations to engage him in sensory, movement, rhythmic, and physical activities to promote physiological states that would shift from his fear-based states (initially immobilized with fear, then alternating between immobilization and mobilization states, with and without fear, as our work together progressed). By restoring his connection to early developmental movements and their associated neurological actions, and varying his moving rhythms in different postures and with a variety of external stimuli, we began to restore his capacity for social engagement. Rather than describe our process, the polyvagal play stations that served as the foundation of our work over 6 months are listed as strategies that any clinician can utilize. We "visited" one to three play stations every session; our sessions changed from weekly to two times per month after 5 months. We worked together a total of 9 months.

Polyvagal play stations are places where children can engage their senses, bodies, movements, and voices in service of shifting physiological states. For Alphonse, who began in a clammed-up, nonverbal immobilized fear state, working nonverbally with BNAs of the developmental progression in movement, facial expressivity, prosody, posture and gaze all served to promote his upregulating to mobilized states (sometimes in fear; sometimes on the edge of fear, in excitement), inching slowly toward brief moments of social engagement. In reflecting on this work, which contributed to the original idea of polyvagal play stations, it became clear that the power of polyvagal-informed DMT to promote social engagement through titrated up-, down-, and side-shifting of physiological state is in the integration of sensory, rhythmic, movement, and, when possible, verbal communication. This integration allows the client and therapist to "hopscotch" between immobilization and mobilization and move between fear and excitement on the pathway to social engagement.

The polyvagal play stations can promote up-, down-, and side-shifting of energy appropriate to the environment, so that children restore their ability to have accurate neuroception, modulate their energy, and begin to regulate their emotions. The physicality of these activities promotes physiological state shifts as the basis for the ability to establish self-regulation.

The polyvagal play stations include:

1. *Rest and settle.* Create a "nest" of soft mats and blankets; include earplugs and eye masks if appropriate. It's also possible to include soothing music if the play station is separate enough from play station #3. Sometimes, I also include a sacral wedge to promote sacral neutral, and therefore vagal tone.

2. *Prop shop.* Have a station with stretch bands, physio-balls, balance boards, and similar items. Playing with these props can promote changes in movement repertoire, feedback through rhythmic activities, and sensory input. By adding music, rhythmic feedback loops that shift body prosody and expressivity (facial and whole-body expressivity) are stimulated, as well as progression through horizontal and vertical postures; balance in muscular tonicity and spinal movements that

support flexion, extension, and dimensional sacral movement are also promoted.

3. *Music:*

a. Have a music station with preselected, culturally appropriate music. Provide high-quality earphones to minimize outside distraction. Encourage either resting or moving/dancing to the music. Have music selections of varying rhythms (slow/fast, heavy/light, tight/loose) to offer a variety of up-, down-, and side-shifting auditory feedback.

b. Have a station with culturally appropriate or familiar and easy to play instruments makers such as rain sticks, chimes, or singing bowls. Choose calming and soothing sounds. Individually or in pairs, play the sounds near (not too near!) the ears to stimulate the social nervous system. Therapist and child can alternate playing together, mirroring (call and response), and "sound conversations" (attuning through sound and music by responding to each other's sounds with a new sound). Working in pairs promotes social connection, relationship, and reciprocity.

4. *Scarves.* Playing with scarves promotes moving, dancing, swaying, rocking, tossing, floating, "flying," and other movement-shaping activities in a way that engages most or all of the body. It expands body repertoire and prosody. Scarves can ignite the imagination, linking present body experience and play to the symbolic realm of language, which "sits" between movement as primary language and spoken word. Depending on a child's age, encourage movements that mimic animals or images from nature, or use the scarves as tactile stimulus to invite self-soothing and regulation. Older children can learn to verbalize their experience.

5. *Chocolate.* The vagus nerve enervates the majority of muscles associated with the larynx and pharynx and the soft palate. Placing small chocolate squares in the mouth and melting them into the roof of the mouth seems to soften the muscles of the spine and increase fluid movement through downregulating the nervous system (or stimulating the parasympathetic). If children do not like or cannot eat chocolate, a culturally appropriate sweet or snack that melts can be substituted.

6. *Sensory station.* Fill a station with a variety of textured objects to stimulate feedback loops associated with touch, which is related to

early co-regulation of the nervous system by caregivers. Other senses can be incorporated just as chocolate incorporates taste (i.e., color for sight, music for auditory, essential oils for olfactory).

7. *Bubble-blowing station.* Blowing bubbles invites play, which is mobilization without fear! It also engages cranial nerves V and VII, part of the Social Engagement System. Following bubbles can engage cranial nerves IX, X, and XI through orienting movements of the neck and head. Having a variety of bubbles (e.g., everything from old-fashioned small bottles to large bubble makers) can invite ranges of expressivity and mouth movement, which can restore social engagement through gradual movement-inspired state shifting.

8. *Polyvagal "balloon buddies."* Polyvagal balloon buddies grew out of this clinical work. I use balloons and magic markers and invite children to draw a picture, symbol, or face on the balloon. Then we begin to blow the balloon up, and make faces in response to the changing shapes on the balloon. This can engage the Social Engagement System and invite playfulness, laughter, and social engagement. (Note: it's important to have agreements around not allowing balloons to pop, and not letting the air out too fast, which creates a noise that can be distressing.)

There is no end to the possibilities for polyvagal play stations. I have used these in one room, with one or a few children; I have created polyvagal play stations in a series of rooms for a group of children. It's important to establish children's abilities to regulate their body responses and determine how much support they need while moving through the stations. Activities that promote up-, down-, and side-shifting, and therefore physiological state shifts, can sometimes promote fear from the unexpected.

Discussion

I did not begin these explorations with Alphonse until 12 weeks into therapy. It will vary based on a child's resources and therapeutic alliance. These play stations formed the bulk of our work together for 6 more months, and in that time, Alphonse increased vertical posture and movement explorations (i.e., he walked, and sometimes even danced, more), so that his movement repertoire increased visibly, as did his kinesphere. As his vocalizations became more frequent and prosodic, and his gaze and facial expressivity slowly returned, he talked a little more. We mostly talked about good things he remembered; there were a few times, from the safety of his hiding place with one of the props nearby, he mentioned seeing blood when people lost limbs, or referred to "bad men who hurt people." When I pressed him to say more, he often clammed up again. Returning to one of the polyvagal play stations would promote a return to movement, interaction, and communication. Although he never fully shared his trauma experience, I believe this work served as a powerful resource for him to begin to reconnect to his body and to early benevolent memories that preceded the war. Because of his age during the war, his memory was predominantly sensorimotoric and image based (Herman, 1997; Rothschild, 2000; Terr, 1990; van der Kolk, 1994, 2014; van der Kolk et al., 2001). Alphonse's dissociated retreat into a silent, nonengaged world was how he survived the horrors he witnessed. Recognizing the brilliance of the body's primitive behavioral strategies in the face of such horror, polyvagal-inspired DMT allowed us to weave threads of connection and coherence between his body and his emotions. We began with early developmental movements, and then journeyed through sensory, rhythmic, movement, and sound-based polyvagal play stations until he was able to socially engage enough to begin communicating. Alphonse needed to experience the somatic foundations of his early development to begin to reconnect to language and to the narrative of his brief life story.

CONCLUSION

The polyvagal theory provides scientific rationale for the use of nonverbal, physiologically based dance, movement, rhythm, and sensorimotoric interventions with survivors of traumatic experience. With children who have not yet developed the full capacity to communicate their inner experience in a coherent, chronological narrative in support of meaning making and well-being, movement-based interventions address the neurological underpinnings of thoughts, feelings, behaviors, and actions. Polyvagal-informed DMT bridges scientific evidence and creative movement as a primary and fundamental pathway to restoring communication, expression, healthy relationship, and a sense of well-being at a crucial stage of one's life. It is necessary for all survivors of trauma, who continue to live in fear, to shift physiological states and restore core rhythmicity in order to experience emotional and psychological well-being. For children, this is especially true. For children who have shut down and withdrawn from caregiving relationships and normal social activity and development, the polyvagal theory provides a deeper understanding of the power of movement and dance in a child's ability, and birthright, to reengage with the world.

FIVE RECOMMENDED PRACTICES

1. Create a safe environment. The cues of safety and danger that we detect influence *how we will move* in an environment. Simple, clean, uncluttered spaces with just enough props, color, art, and beauty can calm the nervous system and invoke socially engaged, play, or rest and settle states. The acoustic environment should not be too loud, and is more likely to promote safety when low-frequency sounds are minimized. Having places where children can hide, rest, play, create, and move can support them to both regulate and shift their physiological states.

2. Speak or sing "prosodically." Often, therapists talk in a slight monotone, attempting to sound calming or soothing. Using a prosodic voice can communicate safety to clients. Inviting clients to practice their own prosody will promote their social engagement behaviors. Even if children don't or won't talk, using a prosodic voice will promote regulation and calm physiological state (i.e., increase vagal tone) by stimulating your and the client's social nervous systems.

3. Make faces! Funny faces, expressive faces, kind faces, animated faces, compassionate faces. Facial expression, similar to prosodic voice, triggers a response in the client that functions as a "neural" exercise of the social engagement system. Meeting a client's gaze in a "soft," nonintrusive manner (if culturally appropriate to make eye contact) can stimulate one of the "rules of social engagement" (gaze). For children who are shut down and will not engage verbally, making faces can foster a connection and "move" them from immobilized to more socially engaged states. At times, animated facial expressions are too stimulating or inappropriate. In these situations, use of a compassionate, soft-gaze facial expression that communicates kindness and caring may shift fear states to states that approximate love, reciprocity, and connection.

4. Change posture. Therapy does not have to take place on a couch, or in a chair, or even sitting in one place on the floor—especially with children who clam up. Sacral neutral promotes vagal tone; posture changes (i.e., stand up, sit down, sit, lie, roll on the floor) can promote sacral movement (flexion and extension, as well as more dimensional wheel-like movements), which may also promote vagal

(continued)

FIVE RECOMMENDED PRACTICES (continued)

tone. If children are posturally withdrawn, mirror their posture and then gently attune by beginning to move just enough to be noticeable, encouraging them to join you in movement. Small movements can lead to bigger, more diverse movements, which promotes playful exploration, plasticity, and social engagement.

5. Move your body and invite your clients to move theirs. Quality of movement and willingness to move—the primary language of connection for humans—will encourage reticent children to move. It is virtually impossible to psychologically shut down or dissociate when we are moving, because moving shifts our physiological state to support the metabolic demands of movement. Taking a walk, doing a 1-minute dance party, or having a stretch time or "shake if off" dance are all ways to promote integration of the body and mind. The effectiveness of movement on expanding the neural pathways between brain and body is optimized when movement is reciprocal and occurs in a context of safety.

REFERENCES

American Dance Therapy Association. (2015). *http://adta.org/*

Bainbridge Cohen, B. (2012). *Sensing, feeling and action: The experiential anatomy of body–mind centering.* Toronto: Contact Editions.

Berrol, C. (1992). The neurophysiologic basis of the mind/body connection in dance/movement therapy. *American Journal of Dance Therapy, 14*(1), 19–29.

Chaiklin, S., Lohn, A., & Sandel, S. (1993). *Foundations of dance/movement therapy: The life and work of Marian Chace.* Columbia, MD: Marian Chace Memorial Fund of the American Dance Therapy Association.

Cottingham, J., Porges, S., & Lyons, T. (1988). Effects of soft tissue mobilization (Rolfing pelvic life) on parasympathetic tone in two age groups. *Journal of American Physical Therapy, 68*(3), 352–356.

Geller, S. M., & Porges, S. W. (2014). Therapeutic presence: Neurophysiological mechanisms mediating feeling safe in therapeutic relationships. *Journal of Psychotherapy Integration, 24*(3), 178–192.

Gray, A. (2015). Dance/movement therapy with refugee and survivor children: A healing pathway is a creative process. In C. Malchiodi (Ed.), *Creative interventions with traumatized children* (2nd ed., pp. 169–190). New York: Guilford Press.

Gray, A. E. (2015). The broken body: Somatic perspectives on surviving torture. In S. L. Brooke & C. E. Myers (Eds.), *Therapists creating a cultural tapestry: Using the creative therapies across cultures* (pp. 170–190). Springfield, IL: Charles C Thomas.

Harrison, B. (2015, September 18). *Embodying ethics: Body–mind tools for creating an ethical practice* [PowerPoint presentation].

Herman, J. (1997). *Trauma and recovery.* New York: Basic Books.

Jackson, H. H. (1882). On some implications of dissolution of the nervous system. *Medical Press and Circular, 2,* 411–414.

Kornblum, R., & Halsten, R. L. (2006). School dance movement therapy for traumatized children. In S. Brooke (Ed.), *Creative arts therapies manual: A guide to the history, theoretical approaches, assessment, and work with special populations of art, play, dance, music, drama, and poetry therapies* (pp. 144–155) Springfield, IL: Charles C Thomas.

Levy, F. (2005). *Dance/movement therapy: A healing art.* Reston, VA: National Dance Association and American Alliance for Health, Physical Education, Recreation, and Dance.

Maslow, A. H. (1943). A theory of human motivation. *Psychological Review, 50*(4), 370–396.

Porges, S. W. (1995). Orienting in a defensive world: Mammalian modifications of our evolutionary heritage: A Polyvagal Theory. *Psychophysiology, 32,* 301–318.

Porges, S. W. (2004). Neuroception: A subconscious system for detecting threats and safety. *Zero to Three, 24*(5), 19–24.

Porges, S. W. (2007). The polyvagal perspective. *Biological Psychology, 74,* 116–143.

Porges, S. W. (2009). The polyvagal theory: New insights into adaptive reactions of the autonomic nervous system. *Cleveland Clinic Journal of Medicine, 76,* S86–S90.

Porges, S. (2011). *The polyvagal theory: Neurophysiological foundations of emotions, attachment, communication, self-regulation.* New York: Norton.

Rothschild, B. (2000). *The body remembers: The psychophysiology of trauma and trauma treatment.* New York: Norton.

Siegel, D. (2012). *The developing mind.* New York: Guilford Press.

Terr, L. (1990). *Too scared to cry.* New York: Basic Books.

van der Kolk, B. (1994). The body keeps the score: Memory and the evolving psychobiology of posttraumatic stress. *Harvard Review of Psychiatry, 1*(5), 253–265.

van der Kolk, B. (2002). The assessment and treatment of complex PTSD. In R. Yehuda (Ed.), *Treating trauma survivors with PTSD* (pp. 127–156). Arlington, VA: American Psychiatric Press.

van der Kolk, B. (2014). *The body keeps the score: Brain, mind and body in the healing of trauma.* New York: Random House.

van der Kolk, B., Hopper, J. W., & Osterman, J. E. (2001). Exploring the nature of traumatic memory: Combining clinical knowledge with laboratory science. In J. J. Freyd & A. P. DePrince (Eds.), *Trauma and cognitive science: A meeting of minds, science and human experience* (pp. 9–31). Binghamton, NY: Haworth Press.

Van Koningsveld, S. R. (2011). Effort and personality According to Rudolf Laban: An artistic inquiry of mobile state. *Dance/Movement Therapy and Counseling Theses*. Paper 1.

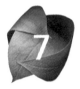

Play Therapy through the Lens of Interpersonal Neurobiology

Up and Over the Mountain

Theresa Kestly

George[1] was clear at his fifth session that he really didn't want to be in my play therapy room. Sullen, with downcast eyes, he came in literally dragging his feet. Without saying a word to me, not even responding when I cheerfully said, "Hello, I'm happy to see you," he went to the shelf of art supplies, chose a large piece of paper, and sat down at the table with the markers. He picked a black marker and drew the outline of a house filling half of the paper. George then proceeded in a laborious manner to color in the outline with a red marker. He used only these two colors for the entire session—black and red (Figure 7.1). He was not going to give any more than that, and he certainly was not going to talk.

George was 8 years old. His mother brought him to play therapy because school officials were threatening to expel him for defiant and aggressive behavior toward his teacher. George had shoved a desk toward her and then slammed the door of his classroom in her face when she tried to correct his behavior. The parents were desperate.

Frankly, I was desperate too. This was our fifth session, and I was beginning to question my skills as a child therapist. I was still somewhat

---

[1]The clinical examples in this chapter are based on composite material drawn from a number of individual cases. I have done it this way to protect confidentiality of patients while preserving authenticity of case examples.

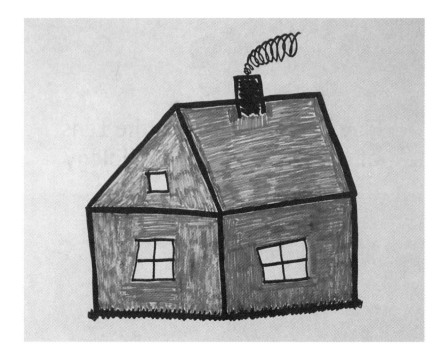

FIGURE 7.1. Black and red house by George.

inexperienced as a play therapist, but until I met George, I had been fairly successful in helping children to engage. George was different, and I felt lost despite the fact that I had created a welcoming and inviting playroom with plenty of nonverbal activities available. During these first five sessions, I tried everything that I had been trained to do. I reflected as well as I could, not knowing exactly what I was reflecting since verbally George was pretty shut down. Whenever I attempted to say anything, he gave no response, not even eye contact or any visible movement that would let me know he had heard me.

In retrospect, I know now that it would have been very helpful when I was struggling with George if I had been able to look at the situation through the lens of interpersonal neurobiology[2] (IPNB), a

---

[2]Siegel (2012a) defines this term in the *Pocket Guide to Interpersonal Neurobiology* as "a consilient field that embraces all branches of science as it seeks the common, universal findings across independent ways of knowing in order to expand our understanding of the mind and well-being. Sometimes abbreviated as IPNB, this field explores the ways in which relationships and the brain interact to shape our mental lives. IPNB is meant to convey the embracing of everything in life from society (interpersonal) to synapses (neurobiology)" (p. AI–42).

cross-disciplinary field grounded in science that explores how we shape one another's brains throughout the lifespan. It would have informed my therapeutic decisions, and I would have been able to address several problems immediately. I had met George before the "decade of the brain" (the period from the mid-1990s to the middle of the 2000s), so I didn't have the benefit of that framework. Although I have never seen another child just like George since that time, I have encountered numerous other children who also just "clam up" when they come into the playroom. They are silent for a number of reasons, but I have come to consistently rely on the IPNB framework when I meet these special youngsters.

In this chapter, I explore several ideas within the framework of IPNB to help formulate ways to work with children who clam up. As play therapists, we have always known intuitively, and from a research perspective, just how important the therapeutic relationship is. Garry Landreth (2012) expressed it beautifully in his seminal book, *Play Therapy: The Art of the Relationship*. We have built our expertise on this core idea. As neuroscience has revealed over the past two decades, we are beginning to understand more deeply why the therapeutic relationship is so crucial to healing brains and lives wounded by painful and frightening experiences. The research is showing us that "interpersonal" and "neurobiology" are inextricably bound. In a practical sense, how does an understanding of neurobiology make a difference in the interpersonal relationships of our play therapy? What difference would an IPNB perspective have made when I was struggling to figure out how to reach George?

Daniel Siegel (2012a) talks and writes about the "neurobiology of we" to explain how the concepts of "me" and "we" emerge from how our relationships influence the functioning of our brains. To embark on this journey into the "we" and "me" of neurobiology, we need to navigate, through some interesting discoveries: (1) the polyvagal theory (Porges, 2011); (2) the window of tolerance, a concept introduced by Siegel (2012b); and (3) the PLAY circuitry of the brain (Panksepp & Biven, 2012). How do these concepts come together in a play therapy setting to help us know what to do when we are with children who clam up?

OUR NERVOUS SYSTEM PROTECTS US

The polyvagal theory (Porges, 2011) immediately shifts my view of children who come in with difficulty engaging. Instead of experiencing frustration, these insights help me feel a deep appreciation for their remarkable adaptability in managing threat in their environments. This sense of danger may be coming from the outside world in this moment or from old memories of frightening experiences that are arising now because their relationship with me is new. Whatever the cause, they are experiencing it as real in this moment. As I learn more of children's histories, I can now see that any refusal to connect with me is an automatic response of their nervous system. Porges's theory essentially tells us that children who have experienced neglect, abuse, or trauma have learned that it is not safe to get close to other human beings, making it almost impossible for them to enter fully into the experience of connection and relatedness in healthy ways.

Thanks to Porges's work, when I met 5-year-old Alex, another child from my play therapy practice, I could assume he had good reasons for keeping his distance from almost everyone outside his family, even though I didn't yet know what those reasons might be. He was diagnosed as a *selective mute*[3] during his first year in preschool, just after his third birthday. At home he was very talkative, but at school he simply clammed up. He was also silent when he came into my playroom. Prior to Alex's first session, I learned from his parents that Alex's kindergarten year had been difficult for all of them. The parents said they experienced pain as they watched his anxious reactions to the morning routine of getting ready for school. Alex would begin to withdraw from conversation, and then appear to be confused about what was expected of him in the small tasks of getting dressed and brushing his teeth. His mother, Mrs. Wilson, said that when they told him it was time to get into the car to go to school, his body would stiffen and then stay that way during the entire 10-minute drive. He would still be that way when she left him at his classroom door. She could only assume that he must have experienced this bodily rigidity all day long.

Mrs. Wilson's description of Alex's *stiff-as-a-board* bodily state fit well with my first impression of Alex when he came into the waiting room, partially hiding behind his mother, looking down at the floor. When I softly said, "Hi, Alex," he turned his head slightly away without responding. By this time, I had begun to use the IPNB framework to make clinical decisions, and from the intake interview with his parents, I already knew that Alex's nervous system had been stretched to the limit with relationships that felt unsafe to him, and I knew that it would be important not to move too quickly.

Porges's polyvagal theory was helpful to me, not only to inform my clinical decisions in how to relate to Alex, but also to provide his parents with a clear explanation of what might be happening within their son. Using these theoretical ideas, we were able to talk more easily about therapeutic goals and about what they could do to speed Alex's recovery.

---

[3] *Selective mutism* is a psychiatric disorder in which a person who is normally capable of speech is unable or unwilling to speak in certain situations or to specific people.

As I often do in these situations, I referenced the work of Porges to introduce them to the core idea of how children play within safe relationships, building resilience and communication skills through co-regulating with the therapist. I can share how new neural pathways are built in this relationship so that the world feels safe enough to engage again.

THE TRAFFIC LIGHT ANALOGY

Porges and Carter (2010) use a traffic light analogy to help explain the polyvagal theory, and I often share a visual of it with children and adults to help them appreciate the extraordinary adaptability of their nervous systems. It seems to comfort them to know they have an inner intelligence that has been keeping them safe. Porges (2011) coined the term *neuroception*[4] to describe the ability of our nervous system to detect threat or safety well below the level of conscious awareness, and then adaptively adjust our behaviors. Let's look at the traffic light analogy in Figure 7.2 to understand part of the reasons why children clam up.

As we approach a traffic light, we usually hope for green. Green signals that we are safe to move ahead. We mammals prefer this branch of our nervous system—the social engagement branch, also called the ventral vagal parasympathetic branch. In the figure of the traffic light, we can see that this is the zone where we feel safe—where we can use face-to-face communications and vocal sounds to signal to others that it is okay to approach, that we can come together and settle in to relax, enjoy ourselves, or even comfort each other. In this branch, we are cognitively at our best because our ears are tuned to be able to easily take in the meaning of words that are being spoken to us.

If we neuroceive (automatic detection of safety or threat) that something in our internal or external environment is not safe, we automatically move out of the social engagement system into the yellow zone—caution, or the sympathetic branch of our nervous system. This branch helps us to mobilize so we can fight or flee, but our cognitive abilities diminish because we need to focus exclusively on the source of the threat. Our ears are also tuned to the larger environment so we can hear sounds of danger (low pounding or high screeching sounds), at the expense of being able to hear human voices clearly. We may feel heightened arousal, increasing heart rate, and an urge to move.

---

[4]Porges and Carter (2010) define *neuroception* as the detection of features seen in others or the environment—without awareness—that dampens defensive systems and facilitates social behaviors or promotes defensive strategies of mobilization (fight–flight) *or* immobilization (shutdown, collapse, dissociation).

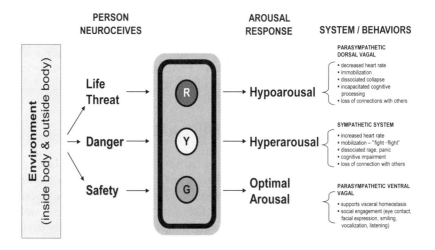

FIGURE 7.2. Autonomic nervous system traffic light analogy. Based on Porges (2011), Porges and Carter (2010), and Kestly (2014). Copyright ©2016 by Theresa Kestly. Reprinted with permission from the author. All rights reserved.

If we begin to have a neuroception of helplessness, it is no longer possible to take action in our defense, so a red light comes on in our nervous system as we enter the dorsal vagal parasympathetic branch of our nervous system. It is a state of hypoarousal—a shutting down where the heart and other organs of the body literally slow down, and we experience immobilization that sometimes causes us to faint or to dissociate and collapse, feigning or actually preparing for death. While cognitive abilities are seriously diminished, and sometimes even obliterated in this branch, there is an underlying motivation to stay safe by being so still that we may go unnoticed, or so submissive that we will no longer be hurt. In this state, there is also a release of endorphins to diminish the pain we might experience in dying.

In essence, our polyvagal system is helping us decide how close or how far away we need to be in relationship with others. With Alex, I could put this knowledge to work right away. I knew from my first encounter with him that his sympathetic system was highly aroused by meeting yet another stranger. His nervous system was protecting him with his urge to flee (visible to me as he turned his head away when I greeted him). He was managing the high arousal by shutting down my attempt to connect. I knew then that it would be important to have

Alex's mother or father in the playroom at least for our first few sessions while he and I developed our own dance of safety. During our intake session, I had prepared Mr. and Mrs. Wilson for this possibility so that they could join my efforts to cultivate safety by avoiding any attempts to get Alex to talk.

While talking with the Wilsons, I shared an analogy from Siegel and Hartzell (2003) that talks about the idea of the accelerator and brakes of a vehicle to explain how we use the prefrontal region of our brains to regulate this emotional energy that flows through our autonomic nervous systems. The accelerator (sympathetic system) increases arousal, speeding up our hearts and sending a message to our brains that we need to mobilize (fight–flight). The braking (parasympathetic system) slows our hearts in two different ways. One way is the calm we experience when we feel safe and are using our social engagement systems (ventral vagal) to connect with others. The other braking function happens when we experience life-threatening situations that cause our dorsal vagal parasympathetic system to help us protect ourselves by shutting down, dissociating, or collapsing. The prefrontal region is strategically located in the brain, where it directly connects the three major areas that coordinate to help us regulate our emotions and impulses: (1) the neocortex (necessary for reasoning, complex thinking, empathic connection, and emotion regulation), (2) the limbic system (motivational and emotional processing, also the home of unresolved trauma), and (3) the brainstem (bringing in input from the body). I shared that when there have been fearful or painful experiences that haven't been resolved, the connections between these parts could not be built, so we remain vulnerable to these implicit memories coming into our daily lives in ways that frighten us. We imagined that Alex's inability to speak outside his safe home was a result of some buried memories that he and I could explore and integrate through playing together.

THE OPTIMAL AROUSAL OF PLAY

When I show parents the visual of the traffic light analogy, I usually show them a second handout, Figure 7.3, to help them see the optimal ebb and flow of the arousal system (shown here as a solid line in the form of a wave within the window) when we are operating in the social engagement branch (ventral vagal) of our nervous systems. This ventral vagal branch is placed in the middle to show the ups and downs of optimal regulation in comparison to the overly high-arousal (sympathetic) and overly low-arousal (dorsal vagal parasympathetic) branches. Siegel

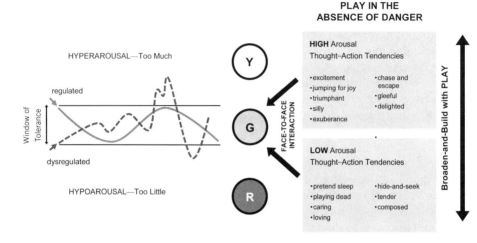

FIGURE 7.3. Optimal arousal compared to hyperarousal and hypoarousal. Based on Porges (2011, 2012), Porges and Carter (2010), and Kestly (2014). Copyright ©2015 by Theresa Kestly. Reprinted with permission from the author. All rights reserved.

(2012b) refers to this optimal zone as our *window of tolerance.*[5] The broken line that begins at the bottom of the window of tolerance shows a dysregulated nervous system that goes outside the window of tolerance with too much or too little arousal. As Siegel (2012b) suggests, behavior outside the window may easily lead to chaos or rigidity. Trauma can make this window very narrow, causing people to react to many small triggers in an attempt to stay safe as they neuroceive danger. The traffic light analogy is carried over into this figure with the three circles indicating R (red), Y (yellow), and G (green) to remind us that the social engagement system is like having a green light, and the yellow and red are indicating escalating threat with corresponding shifts in levels of arousal in the nervous system.

As we will see in the course of Alex's therapy, the right side of Figure 7.3 shows how play therapy helps children to develop resilience as explained by the broaden-and-build theory of Fredrickson (Fredrickson 2009, 2013; Kok & Fredrickson, 2010). Integrating her concepts with

---

[5]Siegel (2012a) defines *window of tolerance* as "a span of tolerable levels of arousal in which internal or external stimuli can be processed in a flexible and adaptive manner. Outside of the window for this particular state, the individual moves toward chaos or toward rigidity of response" (p. AI–84).

the polyvagal theory of Porges, we can see in the diagram that positive high-arousal and positive low-arousal emotions help us to develop a repertoire of behaviors that broaden rather than narrow our options as our nervous system responds to stimuli from the environment. We do this by experiencing low- and high-arousal positive emotions in the absence of danger, and thus, as Porges says, we co-opt the sympathetic (yellow) and the dorsal vagal (red) in the service of the ventral vagal (green). Usually we think of the yellow and red zones as negative because they easily lead to chaotic or rigid behaviors, but in the case of play that is occurring in the absence of danger, the nervous system is learning to manage high and low states of arousal in a positive way, leading to a broader repertoire of behaviors. This is possible through face-to-face interactions because we are constantly assessing the intentions of others in play relationships through visual cues. The face is a portal to the nervous system because the vagus nerve is entangled with the striated muscles of the face. When we have a neuroception of safety, our faces are very mobile, and as threat arrives and escalates, our faces become more and more immobile, beginning with the forehead. In this way, we are in constant visual communication with one another about how safe or dangerous we believe the world to be in this moment. We will return to this discussion when we introduce Porges's polyvagal definition of play.

When I showed this handout to the Wilsons, we talked about how play helps children gradually increase the intensity of emotions they can experience while staying connected with us, and how we as parents and therapists can help them to manage the over- and underarousal by being present in the play and providing repair when we sense that children have exceeded what they can manage in terms of the optimal zone. Part of the task of parenting and of therapeutic intervention in play therapy is to widen this window through co-regulation. We can do this by watching the facial and head signals that tell us when the boundaries of the window have been exceeded so that we can offer repair. I shared several examples of infant–parent play with the Wilsons, such as peek-a-boo, to illustrate how this co-regulation develops quite naturally during early infancy. As parents, we usually don't have to think about it too much. Both parents fondly recalled the silly games they used to play with Alex during his first years. I told them that we could build on these patterns of co-regulating play in age-appropriate ways to help Alex widen his window of tolerance, thus helping to restore his access to his social engagement system.

I prepared the Wilsons for participation in Alex's beginning play sessions. I asked them to follow my lead in the playroom in terms of putting no pressure on Alex to do or say anything. This kind of nonjudgmental receptivity is at the heart of safety. I showed the parents the

playroom during our intake session, and I told them that it was specifically designed with a variety of play modalities to give children a wide
range of possible activities. I speculated that something would attract
Alex's attention and we would begin with that. I told the parents that
I would model how to reflect whatever he was able and willing to give
us. I asked them specifically not to correct any of his behaviors in the
playroom; I explained that this was only for the time that they were with
Alex in the playroom. Some parents have difficulty with this permissiveness of the playroom because they fear they will lose control over
their children outside the playroom, and so I am careful to tell parents
how it is linked to our goals for therapy. Tying the permissiveness to the
safety of the nervous system helps them to make sense of the strategy. I
also explain that I fully support their parental tasks of guiding and correcting their children's behavior outside of the playroom, and how this
practice with reflecting will actually help them do that. We make a clear
distinction between what needs to happen within the limits of the special playtime and what happens in ordinary daily routines. I assured the
parents that we would work on the distinction of moving into and out of
the permissiveness of special playtime with Alex. What I say to the child
when I introduce the playroom usually helps parents to understand. It
goes something like this: "This is our special playroom. In here you can
do almost anything you like, and if there is something that you can't do,
I'll let you know right away." When I used these words to introduce Alex
to the playroom in his first session, he looked at his mother. She smiled,
put her arm over his shoulder and said, "Oh, so many choices." He was
tentative, but he looked around, and I could see the tension in his body
ease just a little. He walked over to the shelf where the toy trains were
and picked up Thomas the Tank Engine. He put it on the floor, picked
several more cars and hooked them together.

I waited, and as I did, I took several long deep breaths, being mindful of my own sense of being present with Alex and his mother. From
IPNB I knew that my inner state of regulation, whether or not I felt
anchored primarily in the calm of my own social engagement system,
would be felt by his system through the resonance circuitry that allows
us to shape one another's brains and experience, again below the level
of conscious awareness. As I remained in ventral vagal, or consciously
returned to it when it slipped away through mindful awareness, Alex's
brain would begin to rewire in patterns more similar to mine so that
he would gradually gain more access to his social engagement system.
Research on our attachment system (Badenoch, 2008; Siegel, 2012b;
Schore, 2012; Stern, 1997) makes it clear that children's ability to manage the arousal of their nervous system depends on the co-regulation
that develops within safe, caring relationships. Restoring Alex's sense of
safety through our co-regulation would be essential in his therapy.

Alex's refusal to talk at school was puzzling to his parents and to me, except for the fact that they were aware that Alex had previously experienced a lot of stress in response to an unpleasant preschool teacher. However, they had been very supportive of his distress, so it seemed unlikely that was enough for him to go silent. At the beginning of Alex's therapy, I had conducted a thorough parent interview, and I listened carefully as they told me about his adoption at 6 months of age. He had been removed from his biological parents at 3 months of age and then lived with a foster family until the Wilsons adopted him. Although there were pieces of missing information, generally I learned that the adoption had gone smoothly. The Wilsons were highly invested in caring for Alex, and from their description, it seemed that the attachment process had gone well. There were some medical interventions at age 2½, when Alex had to have an MRI because of an unexplained seizure. The father, an emergency medical technician, had good information about the procedure, and he felt that Alex had handled it pretty well. Apart from the very early months of his life, there was nothing obvious in the intake interview that could explain Alex's reluctance to talk at school or to be wary of people outside his family. I did take note of the MRI as a possible traumatic experience, but it seemed that the situation had been handled as well as could be expected. We would simply need to wait for the nonverbal storytelling of Alex's play to learn why he was clamming up at school. More important, I believed that his play would lead us to the joint experiences that would allow him to revise his implicit expectation that the world is mostly unsafe. Through our co-regulating joint play, the neural wiring holding this expectation would gradually be reshaped toward anticipating relationships to be more like what he and I were experiencing together—safe, warm, supportive.

THE BRAIN CIRCUITRY OF PLAY

As I mentioned above, another researcher, Jaak Panksepp (Panksepp & Biven, 2012) has contributed to my understanding of how play heals brains. His discovery of seven emotional–motivational systems buried deep in our midbrain helps us picture how playing together makes it possible for even traumatic experiences to be rewired. He tells us that the SEEKING[6] system, which guides our urge to move and be curious, is the "granddaddy" of all the rest. When we feel disconnected, the SEEKING system devotes its energies to the circuitries of GRIEF/PANIC/

---

[6]Panksepp used capital letters when he wrote about the seven emotional systems (one of them being PLAY) to remind us that he was referring to one of the specific core circuits identified as being intrinsic to all mammals, not just humans.

SEPARATION DISTRESS, FEAR, and RAGE in an effort to restore connection. Both George and Alex exhibited clear signs of these circuits being active in them. However, when we feel reconnected, the systems of PLAY and CARE become active, and SEEKING is free to move outward and explore. This points us again to the central importance of providing safe connection by receiving children just as they are because this is what opens the door to the possibility of healing play. I know that I can count on these emotional–motivational systems—CARE + PLAY + SEEKING—when I am with children who clam up.[7] If I stay present and connected to the child, these systems will gradually come online automatically, and they will help the child to stay in his or her social engagement branch of the nervous system. My central task is to be present without being overly directive so that together we can support connections between the limbic region of their brains and the prefrontal cortex, particularly the orbitofrontal cortex, to wire in a felt sense of safety that brings an increased window of tolerance for all emotions.

Alex lost no time in using his PLAY and SEEKING systems to construct a sandtray that went right to the heart of his difficulty. Like many 5-year-olds, Alex loved the miniature train set, and he quickly set up tracks and a tunnel for the train. He began pulling the train along the tracks and into the tunnel. The first time Alex played with this theme, I had no way of knowing that he was actually showing us (below the level of conscious awareness) what had created unbearable fear in him, but I trusted his PLAY and SEEKING systems, and I did my part by staying present with him within my CARE system. In his second session, Alex elaborated the train theme, but again his primary play action was pulling the train along the tracks and then into the tunnel. When the train was about halfway into the tunnel, Alex deliberately went to the other side of the tunnel and blocked it with a traffic barrier. The train could not pass through the tunnel. It was stuck!

By the third session, Alex was beginning to say a few words to me, and he was establishing eye contact more frequently. His social engagement system was activating more frequently as he learned to trust our play relationship. I was not urging him to speak, and I believe he could feel my delight in his play activities. At the beginning of this session, I told Alex that we would let his mother take a turn in the waiting room while we played. He did not object. As soon as we entered the playroom, Alex headed directly to the train set and then put it in the sand. He chose other objects to elaborate the scene—a few trees, some buildings, and a few vehicles. Once the scene was set, he again made the train chug along

---

[7]For more details on the seven emotional–motivational systems in the brain, see Kestly (2014), Panksepp (1998), and Panksepp and Biven (2012).

the tracks and into the tunnel. When the engine was inside the tunnel, Alex once again blocked off the other end, this time by scooping sand over the tracks and piling it up so that the train could not get through. He said, "Thomas [the train] is stuck!" I reflected, matching the tone and prosody of his speech. Alex's affect and play actions were pointing to the stuck train theme, and I knew it was important, but I still did not know exactly what he was trying to tell us.

THERAPEUTIC PRESENCE

Although I was curious now about what the stuck train might mean, I knew that the most important thing for me to do was to stay mindfully present so that our play relationship could deepen because I believed that was the best way to help Alex find his own unique way. From an IPNB perspective, I knew that we could rely on his brain's inborn push toward optimal integration (Badenoch, 2008; Siegel, 2012b) to find the means for healing whatever was keeping him silent. From Alex's play actions, we could see that something in the tunnel was keeping the train from moving forward on the tracks that Alex had carefully laid out. He had created the potential for movement, but he seemed to be show-ing me that Thomas was up against some obstacle and that he needed to explore all the options in order to find a way through it. Over the next few sessions, Alex tried many variations (his SEEKING system in action) for Thomas. At one point he wanted his father to come into the playroom to help him pull Thomas in reverse out of the tunnel. Alex hooked up a small chain to the last car and then said, "Dad, help me pull Thomas out." Alex's father made pretend sounds associated with strenu-ous efforts as he joined Alex in an effort to pull the train back out of the tunnel. I watched from the sidelines, but I could feel deeply the intense struggle that Alex and his father were exerting as they pulled the train out of the tunnel, and I could see how important it was for Alex to have his father help him in this task.

Suddenly I got it! The MRI (the tunnel)—Alex had to get himself (as Thomas) out of the tunnel. It was a hunch, of course, but it felt pretty clear to me. Alex had been stuck in an MRI machine without either of his parents present. The machines are noisy and scary, and I believe that Alex would have been frightened by the separation from his parents and would have been desperate to get out so that he could reconnect. Even though his parents had been as supportive as possible afterward, the experience of being alone in the MRI machine seemed to have become embedded as a trauma so that part of Alex remained trapped and feel-ing isolated and unsafe. As it turned out, the only way to get out of an

MRI machine is to reverse the procedure. It made perfect sense for Alex to create these play actions of reversing the train as his brain tried to make sense of a very frightening experience. Not long after his father had joined Alex in pulling the train out of the tunnel with the chain, his mother reported that Alex told them that he had had a dream about a "spooky tunnel," and that he could hear Buster, their family dog, barking. Alex said, "I had to get out of the tunnel so that I could help Buster."

Little by little, I could see that Alex was relaxing in the playroom and that his body was moving more freely. Instead of reluctantly following behind one of his parents as he was arriving for therapy, he was now skipping along the walkway to my waiting room, his arms waving openly and vigorously in rhythm with his skipping. He continued playing with the train and the tunnel with many variations, but always Thomas would get stuck about halfway through. Then one day at the end of a session Alex said, "I need my dad to help me." Dad came into the playroom, and of course the train scene was already in place. Alex said, "Thomas wants to go out the other side and up the mountain. Help me push." Together they pushed, but once again, Thomas got stuck (because Alex closed up the other end of the tunnel). This time Alex hooked up the train to a tractor, and as his father watched, Alex made the tractor pull the train back out of the tunnel. Then he asked his father again to push the train through. Failure again! But Alex was not giving up. He said, "One more time, Dad, help me." Together, they carefully guided Thomas into the tunnel. This time Alex went to the other side of the tunnel and cleared away the small piles of sand and debris that were blocking the other end of the tunnel as his father carefully guided Thomas through and out the other side. In unison Alex and his dad raised their arms in a victory gesture and said, "Yaaaay!" Their laughter and huge smiles said it all.

I never spoke to Alex about my hunch regarding the scary experience in the MRI machine when he was younger, but he created an image in the sandtray many sessions later that confirmed my speculation. Without any trains or tracks, Alex placed the train tunnel in the sand with several trees and a few simple wooden structures. Then he got the play mobile hospital bed and put a patient on it. He placed the hospital bed with the patient just inside the tunnel—looking to me very much like a person being rolled into or out of an MRI machine (Figure 7.4).

Although it is interesting for me as a therapist to understand cognitively the traumatic experiences that cause a person's sympathetic (fight–flight) or dorsal vagal parasympathetic (shut down/collapse) systems to come online, knowledge itself does not heal. If I had been able to put all of these details together into an integrated picture to explain Alex's clamming up at school and also when he first came into my playroom,

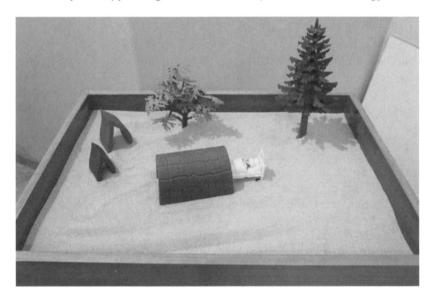

FIGURE 7.4. Alex's tunnel and the hospital patient.

it would not have changed the essential course of our play therapy. Alex would still have needed time to explore and use play actions within a safe relationship where co-regulation could help him have a different experience with his scary MRI tunnel, or as Alex said, "a spooky tunnel." Even when I caught on to his strategy for healing, it would not have been helpful to try to speed up the process by suggesting how he might get Thomas to go through the tunnel. He needed to come to that solution himself so his nervous system and the implicit memory of the MRI could rewire in a pattern that included warm, responsive accompaniment (his father and me) as well as the safety of my CARE system and our PLAY relationship holding all of us in ventral vagal. In Alex's case, he also specifically needed his father's CARE system to be present during his breakthrough. He needed to reconnect with one of his primary attachment figures during his play action related to the traumatic event in the sand.

"I KNEW I COULD, I KNEW I COULD"

Looking back, I have such deep appreciation for how the psyche does its healing work. Alex sensed what he needed to do in his natural desire to move toward wholeness. It was fascinating to watch how his original connection with the *Thomas the Tank Engine* character morphed into something more like *The Little Engine That Could* when he moved from backing out of the MRI tunnel to moving forward in some unique way—up and over the mountain. This experience of breaking free wasn't part of changing the implicit felt sense of the MRI since he never went through that tunnel, but possibly more a metaphor of what comes next after the trauma is integrated. In his sand tray, he built the tracks through and out the other side of the tunnel, thus creating the potential for a breakthrough. As a 2½-year-old, his undeveloped left hemisphere was not capable of making sense of the frightening MRI experience in the absence of his mother and father, but as a 5-year-old, he could make use of play therapy and storytelling to allow him to use both his right and left hemispheres to reprocess the MRI experience in the form of play (in the absence of danger). His use of the familiar *Thomas* story helped his left hemisphere make verbal sense of his experience (the sensations of his implicit memories) of being stuck in a tunnel. His right hemisphere, which specializes in metaphorical thinking, gave him the possibility of finding a positive way to integrate the medical trauma.

As Siegel (2012b) suggests, mental health is a process of integrating the differentiated parts of our brains/minds. The embedded trauma of the MRI experience was disconnected from the flow of his developing brain and left him vulnerable to feelings of danger. We can see how Alex worked on lateral integration (right and left hemispheres), vertical integration (his subcortical motivational systems of PLAY and SEEKING and implicit memory in his limbic system with his prefrontal cortex), and interpersonal integration as Alex returned again and again to my face for reassurance in his trauma play (the co-regulation of me and we) as we played together.

Iain McGilchrist (2009) writes about the relationship of the hemispheres, showing us how the laterality of the brain provides a right-left-right progression that helps us integrate our lived experiences in ever increasing levels of wholeness through metaphorical thinking. In general, our brains experience the world through our senses (seeing, hearing, tasting, smelling, and touching) with the streams of information gathering in our right hemispheres. Then our left hemispheres try to make cognitive sense of these bits and pieces of our experiences. Once this is done, the information is returned to the right hemisphere through the use of metaphor to bring it to a higher level of integration. Alex did not need prompting for this neurobiological right-left-right progression; he simply needed the neuroception of safety provided by deep, caring relationships.

It makes sense that Alex's verbal system would have shut down in the presence of strangers, as his nervous system was trying to protect

him from the threat of being separated from his primary attachment figures during a frightening medical procedure. Exacerbating this response
of his nervous system, Alex's preschool experiences had unfortunately
involved a rather harsh and rigid teacher. It is not at all surprising that
Alex learned to clam up in the presence of strangers, especially at school.

PLAY CO-OPTING THE SYMPATHETIC SYSTEM IN THE ABSENCE OF FEAR

Alex has given us a beautiful illustration of what Porges (2011) has
described as the polyvagal definition of play. Porges tells us how the
PLAY system co-opts the sympathetic nervous system by activating it
and the social engagement system at the same time. He says:

> Play shares with the defensive fight-or-flight behaviors a neurophysiological
> substrate that functionally increases metabolic output by increasing sym-
> pathetic excitation. Concurrent with the sympathetic excitation is a with-
> drawal of the myelinated vagal pathways that characterize the vagal brake.
> Just as the primitive mechanisms mediating immobilization in response to
> life threat can be co-opted to support loving and nutrient processes, so can
> mobilization mechanisms be involved to facilitate both defensive flight-or-
> fight behaviors and pleasurable "play." (p. 276)

Although we usually associate the sympathetic nervous system with
negative feelings (fight–flight), in the case of play the sympathetic nervous system actually helps us to mobilize for the action that is necessary
in play. We can do this because our social engagement system (ventral
vagal branch) is also online, thereby allowing us to check with others
through listening and looking at facial muscles (the smiling of mouth
and eyes) to make sure that we are really "just playing." Alex did frequently check my face for this reason. I noticed it especially as he was
moving Thomas into the tunnel with one hand while closing up the other
end of the tunnel with the other. Thus he was able to manage the high
arousal of the MRI experience as he reconstructed it within the story of
Thomas and our safe play relationship. Looking back at Figure 7.3, we
can see the overlap of the high-arousal thought–action tendencies of the
sympathetic system (yellow) with the calm of the ventral vagal (green).
In this process, the original too-dangerous situation now is held by our
joined windows of tolerance and becomes manageable for his nervous
system. This allows for integration to progressively unfold until he is
on the other side of it and into a new story—up and over the mountain.
    I also believe that Alex used the familiar *Thomas the Tank Engine*

story to manage the experience of collapse that he must have felt when he was wheeled into the MRI machine without his mother or father. Initially he may have wanted to fight or flee, but the instruction was to lie still so that the machine could get a good picture. When he experienced this helplessness, more than likely his dorsal vagal branch (collapse and dissociation) would have come online. Earlier as Alex worked so hard with his father to get through the tunnel, I was reminded of *The Little Engine That Could*. As the little engine struggles to get over the mountain, there are threatening monsters, and at one point, the little engine is buried under a snow avalanche, simulating the collapse and helplessness of the immobilization of the dorsal vagal branch. In this story, however, the little engine prevails by managing these high- and low-arousal events. Again, looking back at Figure 7.3, we can see how play co-opts the low arousal of the dorsal vagal (red) branch, in the absence of danger, to help manage the experience of having positive low-arousal emotions. In this case, there is overlap between the ventral vagal (green) and the dorsal vagal (red) during play. Sometimes moving out of dorsal brings us to the aliveness of sympathetic activation, and as Alex and his father moved out of the tunnel for good, in the safety of play, they could enjoy the deep excitement of this new freedom. This interplay of the three branches of our autonomic nervous system becomes a symphony of healing energies.

The Little Engine That Could ends in victory as the little engine overcomes huge challenges so that he could deliver his gifts to the boys and girls on the other side of the mountain. As he is chugging down the other side of the mountain, the little engine says, "I knew I could, I knew I could, I knew I could." It was beautiful to watch Alex's confidence develop and his window of tolerance widen in response to his playing out his challenging experiences within the safety of our play relationship. As I reflected on how it all unfolded, I could see that even though Alex had repeated the same scene over and over, I was pretty sure this was not *stuck trauma play* because everything else in the scene was being elaborated each time he repeated it, and also because Alex was not doing this play in a vacant, rigid, or dissociated manner. He was vigorous, very connected to the story with each repetition, and he brought all his creative energy to it, including asking for his father's support at crucial moments.

As Alex and I completed our work, I was drawn to reflect on George's silence so many years ago, I can sense how much more closed down he was than Alex, and how his distress was reflected in his outbursts. Picturing the pent-up sympathetic activation behind his inability to engage and his lack of regulation at school, I can now imagine holding his upset within my ventral vagal receptivity until there was sufficient safety for him to become more vulnerable. Just having that picture would have relieved my feelings of desperation. I now understand that George also brought an additional emotional–motivational activation in terms of Panksepp's systems—RAGE—an expression of disconnection with no repair. I am finding that the wisdom offered by Porges and Panksepp consistently quiets my own left-hemisphere questioning about how to help and the anxiety that comes with that, so I am better able to be the receptive container and playmate each child needs.

This is the story of play—how it helps us to prevail in challenging situations, even trauma. Play allows us to visit the high- and low-arousal branches of our nervous systems in the absence of danger. It can help us to expand our windows of tolerance. Where traumatic events create collapse and clamming up, play relationships create the joy that opens us up. Play heals, allowing us to live our lives fully. This is the story of the IPNB of play.

FIVE RECOMMENDED PRACTICES

1. Stay calm in the presence of a child who appears to be disconnecting from a therapeutic relationship.

2. Maintain respect and be curious about the remarkable adaptability of the nervous system to manage threatening situations.

3. Teach parents the core idea that children use play within safe relationships to build resilience and communication skills through learning to manage the arousal levels of their nervous systems.

4. Prepare parents for the possibility of participating in a play session with simple concepts of the interpersonal neurobiology of play (e.g., the nervous system, the PLAY system, the window of tolerance, noticing fight–flight–freeze behaviors).

5. Allow time for children to use the intelligence of their nonverbal right hemispheres to solve problems.

REFERENCES

Badenoch, B. (2008). *Being a brain-wise therapist: A practical guide to interpersonal neurobiology.* New York: Norton.
Fredrickson, B. (2009). *Positivity: Top-notch research reveals the upward spiral that will change your life.* New York: Three Rivers Press.

Fredrickson, B. (2013). *Love 2.0: Creating happiness and health in moments of connection*. New York: Penguin.

Kestly, T. (2014). *The interpersonal neurobiology of play: Brain-building interventions for emotional well-being*. New York: Norton.

Kestly, T. (2015). *Handouts for interpersonal neurobiology*. Unpublished Manuscript, Corrales, NM.

Kok, B., & Fredrickson, B. (2010). Upward spirals of the heart: Autonomic flexibility, as indexed by vagal tone, reciprocally and prospectively predicts positive emotions and social connectedness. *Biological Psychology, 85*(3), 432–436.

Landreth, G. (2012). *Play therapy: The art of the relationship* (3rd ed.). New York: Routledge.

McGilchrist, I. (2009). *The master and his emissary: The divided brain and the making of the Western world*. New Haven, CT: Yale University Press.

Panksepp, J. (1998). *Affective neuroscience: The foundations of human and animal emotions*. New York: Oxford University Press.

Panksepp, J., & Biven, L. (2012). *The archaeology of mind: Neuroevolutionary origins of human emotions*. New York: Norton.

Porges, S. (2011). *The polyvagal theory: Neurophysiological foundations of emotions, attachment, communication, and self-regulation*. New York: Norton.

Porges, S., & Carter, S. (2010). The love code: Social engagement and social bonding. Available at *www.eabp.org/pdf/The_Polyvagal_Theory_S_Porges.pdf*.

Schore, A. N. (2012). *The science of the art of psychotherapy*. New York: Norton.

Siegel, D. (2012a). *Pocket guide to interpersonal neurobiology*. New York: Norton.

Siegel, D. (2012b). *The developing mind: How relationships and the brain interact to shape who we are* (2nd ed.). New York: Guilford Press.

Siegel, D. J., & Hartzell, M. (2003) *Parenting from the inside out*. New York: Penguin Putnam.

Stern, D. (1997). *The first relationship: Infant and mother*. Cambridge, MA: Harvard University Press.

Treating Adolescent Attachment Trauma

Ten Ways to Co-Regulate and Stay Connected

Martha B. Straus

Louisa, age 13, was referred by her beleaguered parents for a con-
stellation of escalating challenges, including school refusal (she was part
way through seventh grade when we met), noncompliance with medication, self-harming tantrums, poor hygiene, head- and stomachaches,
lack of friends, difficulty falling and staying asleep, hoarding food, and
compulsive overeating.

Louisa had been adopted at the age of 3 after experiencing significant early attachment trauma, disruption, and loss. Her adoptive parents were very committed to her and determined to help her overcome
her troubled history. Although Louisa had made progress over the years
(e.g., no longer wetting the bed or requiring supervision in basic self-care),
she continued to experience debilitating emotional, behavioral, learning, and social problems. With the increased expectations and changes
of adolescence, she was falling behind more rapidly. Notably, also, she
harbored a growing awareness of her differences and shortcomings. She
described this succinctly in an early meeting with me, explaining her

unwillingness to go to school: "I'm probably the only adopted and learning disabled kid in my school. I'm fat and wear glasses, and people say horrible things to me." Any motivation Louisa may have had to try to keep up was diminishing as it became harder for her to fit in. Along with a severe reading disability, she was overwhelmed with anxiety and self-doubt during the school day.

Like many teens with attachment trauma, Louisa was easily dys-regulated by seemingly small changes in routine and the challenges of peer interactions. Her large regional junior high school—with daily schedule variations, crowded hallways and classrooms, confusing and dramatic social expectations, and multiple busy teachers—completely overwhelmed her fragile coping resources. Louisa maintained just one tenuous friendship with a similarly marginalized classmate; when they had one of their frequent conflicts, she didn't see any reason to go to school at all.

At times, Louisa could become hyperactivated. She might begin shouting and swearing in outbursts of anger that seemed disproportionate to the provocation. Someone speaking "disrespectfully" to her or chewing loudly after she'd told them to stop, for example, might send her into fits of inexplicable rage. But, as I soon discovered firsthand, she also managed her overwhelming internal world by deactivating; in some stressful situations (including, alas, therapy) Louisa would shut down completely.

I tried to move slowly in the first hours we spent together, as I felt my way into connection with Louisa. I heard about her beloved pets, TV shows she was binge-watching, and even a few hints of her heart-wrenching loneliness. But she was so easily dysregulated that I still had trouble maintaining our connection for a whole therapy hour. She could become extremely irritated with me if I asked too many questions or if I wondered about something too intently, although she wouldn't say so. Inquiring whether I'd annoyed her *really* annoyed her. Once stressed, Louisa might just glower down at her hands as she fiddled with rings or a bracelet, and wait out our time. If she'd had a fight somewhere, or wasn't feeling well, or if we got too close to a stressful topic—or maybe if she was emotionally drained from just holding it together at school all day—she would simply shut her eyes and check out. In the first few months, before we had much of a relationship, I really struggled to get her to reconnect; she'd sit there, glassy eyed for 20 or 30 endless minutes at a stretch, Sphinx-like and mute.

During these dissociative spells, I had time for long inner conversations, debating with myself about whether to keep pushing in one direction or another, to suggest a few grounding techniques, to ask her (fruitlessly) about what was happening in the moment, to open up a few more minutes of room for the silence, to suggest playing a game, to wait patiently, full of unconditional positive regard and a benign expression on my face, or to simply end the session. I tried everything I could think of, to little avail. Louisa didn't know how to use me to stay regulated, or to feel better again. And because it is so hard to stay present with someone this determined to be out of touch, I did my share of mental wandering, too.

Truth told, Louisa had a much vaster array of dissociative strategies than I; once, early on, after yawning and yawning, she closed her eyes, and evidently fell soundly asleep in the session. I simply couldn't rouse her. At the end, I had to get her amused father to come in and give her a gentle shake. She stretched and departed without saying a word. Before the next session, I took the time to reflect and regroup. I now had a sense of how easily she could feel frightened and overwhelmed. I knew I had to find a way to create enough *felt* safety so Louisa might stay regulated and in connection with me more of the time.

Adolescents like Louisa, entering therapy with a history of abuse and neglect, often struggle along every developmental pathway. Their emotional dysregulation—marked by extremes of dissociation and hyperarousal—is connected to other problems regulating themselves physically, behaviorally, cognitively, and socially. And even with multiple supports in place, the legacy of early attachment trauma often continues to shape and define their identity and relationships in essential ways well into adulthood.

Compared to other age groups, traumatized adolescents pose unique challenges for therapy—they may be unable or unwilling to engage in representational play, refuse to comply with CBT-type conversation and homework, lack sufficiently supportive caregivers for family therapy, and are still developmentally unprepared to talk meaningfully about their emotional and physical experience. Like Louisa, they may also be terrified by even the prospect of relationships that might make them vulnerable to rejection and abandonment.

Becoming that safe and reliable adult for a traumatized adolescent is also particularly hard. It can take more time, and often involves greater risk; you may encounter dangerous behaviors not commonly faced in treatment with younger children (e.g., sexual acting out, substance abuse, severe self-harm, delinquency) and higher rates of treatment dropout. The increase in the role and influence of the peer group combined with significantly diminished adult presence outside of the office further distinguishes the singular importance of the therapeutic relationship in work with traumatized adolescents.

TIME IN, NOT TIME OUT

The reflective practice of *time in* describes a strategy for working with traumatized teens using attuned connection with an emotionally regulated therapist as the primary technique. The therapist has to be all in: self-aware, engaged, and compassionate. For me, and most people I know, these vital qualities must be developed and practiced. Since the therapy grows an actual attachment relationship, along with a transferential one, we have to be able to use our *presence* effectively in the service of the treatment. To this end, we must first foster our own capacity to *be present* before we can demand it of a terrified, or furious teen. In other words, to make a difference, we have to really show up.

For a variety of reasons, we're apt to trivialize our importance to adolescents who need us most; we may also minimize our responsibility for their emotional and behavioral regulation. We place so much emphasis on sheer expertise, wanting to believe that these distraught adolescents will feel better if they can just try out a few more self-soothing and problem solving skills. In doing so, we may overlook the bigger mechanism for change: *limbic resonance.* Our fully formed and regulated adult emotional brain soothes their overwrought immature one.

Our default use of "time out," and all the attendant emphasis on teaching self-regulation misses the point with these most vulnerable kids. For traumatized adolescents, time-out often doesn't work (e.g., the problem persists, the behavior resumes immediately, the teen gets more agitated and resentful), and is often even harmful. From the start, like everyone else, these teens first have to learn to rely on others to feel better. Down the road, if they have the capacity to be comforted, and know what it feels like, they can learn to self soothe. Even then, though, in times of greater stress, it still helps to have someone else to lean on—for us all.

In most families, beginning at birth, parents loan babies—and then children, adolescents, *and* emerging adults—their adult regulatory system for a couple dozen years. There are excellent developmental reasons for this. But complexly traumatized teens usually miss out on this opportunity when they're little, and so a major goal of therapy is to provide the experience of successfully depending on someone in order to feel better. In other words, adults—including therapists—need to be regulated themselves in order to help heal attachment trauma. Regulation is modeled, mirrored, supported, felt, and named. When we are reactive to an escalating teen, we feed the fire. When we find ways to stay calmly attuned and connected, we help to quench it. Parents of infants have known this since the beginning of time; now we also have neuroscience and evolutionary biology to explain why (e.g., Siegel, 2012).

Co-regulation isn't just for babies; it's for us all, and perhaps especially it's for traumatized adolescents and their red-hot brains.

For kids like Louisa, it's a gigantic leap to allow someone to provide comfort to them. They don't trust that others are reliable, nor do they believe they merit such care. Their behavior puts to the test the most important question: Will you be there for me when I really need you? When we send them away, or chide them for being irrational, or get upset because *we* can't tolerate what they are doing, or press them to the point of dissociation, our answer is simply, *No*.

Once I realized I'd been flooding Louisa with my eagerness for connection, unintentionally causing her to redouble her efforts to defend herself from me, I pivoted. The next time she came in, and without a barrage of language that she so evidently experienced as threat, I showed Louisa a new 500-piece jigsaw puzzle of horses grazing. (This activity choice was an educated guess; she'd already told me she was a horse and puzzle enthusiast.) I suggested we might do it together over the next few weeks. She shrugged noncommittally, but took the box from me, and went over to the table I'd pointed to. She dumped out the pieces, not bothering to glance at me a second time. But she came back more willingly the next week, if only to work on the puzzle. When we were side by side at the table, I was as calm and engaged with her as I could breathe myself into, trusting the process and my adult limbic brain to bring her into relationship with me, over time. The conversations we had at first were mostly about our shared interest in the puzzle, but we searched *together* for pieces, marveled *together* at our progress, and *together* invited her father to come see our completed masterpiece.

A few weeks in, while we were still doing the puzzle, more amiably, she turned to me, and asked abruptly, "So when are you going to ask me important questions?" I grinned at her and asked, "Like what?" She gave me the eye-roll I came to know well in subsequent years, and replied, "Duh, like about being adopted!" Doing that puzzle early in therapy with Louisa fulfilled a main underlying objective in treating attachment trauma: it provided her with the experience of being in a relationship in a new, more connected, and regulated way.

GOALS OF TREATMENT

Interventions in therapy with traumatized teens can draw from almost every paradigm under the sun, as long as they are offered in the service of these vital goals: feeling safe in relationship; acquiring the hardiness and skills to seek and sustain attachments even in the face of inevitable ruptures; experiencing and recognizing a range of strong and powerful feelings; relying on others to regulate, and then learning to self regulate these feelings; and developing empathy and self-compassion. The only proviso is that the interventions have to make sense for a specific adolescent client, taking into consideration her developmental level as well as her chronological age. This means we might draw cartoons with a 19-year-old or engage in persona/parts work with a 13-year-old.

One of the greatest challenges of adolescent treatment, therefore, is first figuring out trauma's developmental impact, and then resetting the expectations bar as therapy progresses. Two cases come to mind immediately. Sixteen-year-old Max, needing a shave, spent most of our first hour upside-down on the couch passing a cushion from foot to foot, and then lying on the floor building with Legos while we chatted. Twelve-year-old Sophie, tiny as a third grader, crossed her legs, looked right at me and said, "I want to tell you about the crazy dream I had last night." Finding the sweet spot for relationship with these adolescents isn't chronological!

ISOLATION AND CONNECTION

Early attachment trauma taught our teen clients that they couldn't depend on comfort from caregivers who behaved in dangerous and unreliable ways. For many of these adolescents, beginning in infancy, they began to hyperactivate and/or deactivate in the face of interpersonal stress. Such secondary attachment strategies enabled them to survive, but at considerable cost. By the time they arrive at our door, they are not just disconnected from relationships with others, but also from their own internal experiences. They are often called defensive, reluctant, resistant, defiant—or worse; they are seldom motivated to "explore" their feelings about anything, and especially not the trauma.

Indeed, compared to the tsunami of raw emotion they're trying to keep in check, our adolescent clients may have only a few explicit trauma memories to relate. We probably won't have specific events to process with them as in PTSD work. Rather, attachment trauma presents more commonly as overwhelming affect in search of reason. This may help us understand why adolescents' explanations for their dysregulation make so little sense to us. It's likely, for example, that Louisa didn't really have a meltdown simply because her classmate chewed too loudly. Rather, she could have been feeling lonely and anxious in the cafeteria, and become internally flooded. Without self-awareness or a sense of safety, she gave a name to her distress, as plausible as any she might latch onto, as she got buried under the waves.

And we know that isolation—including emotional isolation—is in itself traumatizing for human beings; *our brains actually code it as danger*. Even though we all feel alone some of the time, it seems clear that most psychopathology is associated with the experience of chronic disconnection (e.g., Johnson, 2009; Jordan, 2010). By the time adolescents come into our care, they will likely have endured debilitating experiences of terror and attachment insecurity that are both the cause and effect of their struggles in relationships. The challenge for us, however, is appreciating that this disconnection has also protected them from additional harm; it's likely that previous attempts to be authentic and vulnerable with significant others have resulted in severe emotional pain. Traumatized adolescents, then, come to see us facing a true dilemma: their sense of disconnection is the source of both safety and terrible, soul-sapping loneliness. Following are some practical, evidence-based ways to form and sustain connections with these slow-to-trust teens.

TEN STRATEGIES

Foster Dependence

This therapy relationship is an attachment relationship, and as such it supports the adolescents with a fundamental expectation for *effective* dependence. We want to become more adaptive attachment figures than they have had in the past, helping them *earn* attachment security with us. To this end, we strive to be the most reliable nurturer we can: dependable, attuned, available, forgiving, flexible, and self-aware. We want to help adolescents experience themselves in relation to others in a new way. And we have to try over and over and over again. We're creating new brain circuits to overwrite and add to the old ones, and such integration—implicitly attending to the right hemisphere while engaged in left-hemisphere naming and organizing—takes time. We need to enact dependability until they get it. We say, "Next week, same time"; "You can call or text me if you need me during the week"; "I was thinking about you"; "Here's the poem I was telling you about"; "I'm so glad to see you, I missed you"; "I'm here for you, even if your body is not so sure that's true"; "It looks like you're still feeling a little fragile, can I call you later just to check in?"

Keep It in the Room

Whenever possible, bring the conversation into the present. In this work, we attend most closely to the relational–emotional experiences in the moment, explicitly connecting what's happening with us to their experience of other relationships. We note, for example:

"People made you mad today; am I making you mad?"

"It seems you're expecting me not to understand this since your teacher didn't. I imagine that's pretty frustrating right now."

"I'm feeling confused; are you?"

"What's it like for me to ask you about that?"

"This is hard for us to talk about."

"I'm feeling touched/sad/scared/happy as I hear you say that."

"What happened right now when you laughed at that?"

"I'm here; you are not alone."

"You seem pretty out of sorts today; can I help?"

"I am with you."

"It *is* scary."

"You are safe."

"We're not connecting well right now, and I want to do better."

"That is hilarious; tell me more!"

"What's going on right now?"

"I wonder if you are feeling this, too?"

"I'm so moved that you are able to tell me this."

"Can we just be here now, feet on the ground together?"

"I'm feeling a little worried about you; is it okay if I say so?"

"I think I just missed the boat on that one, I'm so sorry; can we try again?"

Repair Quickly

All therapists, no matter how well trained, how deeply present and compassionate, or how skilled, miss a lot. It is simply impossible to pay attention to and "get" another person all of the time. Fortunately, rupture and conflict are not only inevitable, but they're also crucial to development in therapy. This is not to say you should intentionally show up late or contrive some issue so you can resolve it. No need for that; you *will* screw up, without even trying. The important treatment element here, however, is to acknowledge it when you realize you're not in sync, even if it's minutes or possibly weeks later. Do not hesitate to try and try again, no matter how trivial the lapse might seem to you.

A few years ago, I worked with a young man whom I carelessly addressed by his younger brother's name. (Their names rhymed, so that had happened a lot in his life.) He grimaced when I misspoke, so I knew my error really bothered him, but I let it slide—along with our connection for most of the rest of the session. In my semiaware mind, I thought, *People misspeak; this isn't a big deal.* But for this teen, my slip was still hurtful, perhaps tying into a lifetime of feeling unseen and unimportant. With just a few minutes left to go, I realized I was in a hole, and started to climb out of it. I asked about this, also apologizing for not apologizing sooner. He shrugged but didn't deny being irritated with me. And he remained a little grumpy, but came back the next week to try with me again—which he might not otherwise have done.

The truth is that misattunement is inevitable. And we can take some solace from the work of Ed Tronick and his colleagues, who minutely observed interactions between infants and their mothers. This research demonstrates that even the best parents get it wrong a *lot*—on the first try, they can miss the baby's signals a staggering 70% of the time, and still end up with securely attached kids (Tronick, 2007). As with therapy, the interesting part isn't in the misattunement; it's what happens next. Tronick's studies demonstrated that the infant's emotional regulation was actually *enhanced* by ruptures that were followed by repairs. Babies with this experience develop greater mastery of their dysregulated states and an increased sense of safety and security in relationships. These early missteps and corrections within that dance of attunement generalized to other relationships, too. And of course, sustained intimacy is only possible for people who are capable of resolving inevitable conflict.

But the traumatized teens we treat usually have long histories of rupture without repair. I have been the first adult ever to apologize to most of my clients. They have precious little tolerance for the hard work of trying to make it better. One of the common outcomes of attachment trauma for adolescents is a microscopically short fuse for rejection, disappointment, failure, or emotional abandonment. They experience in their bodies a call for whatever secondary strategies they've developed to regulate in the face of this too-familiar sense of disconnection. This means that the effort to reconnect after a rupture, no matter how small and seemingly inconsequential, is *100% ours to make*. Resolving conflict and reattuning are essential to this work, so we need to face disconnection when we feel or know it happened.

We say, "I shouldn't have interrupted you"; "It wasn't respectful of me to keep you waiting"; "I'm really struggling here, and I can tell I'm not getting it at all"; "I'm so grateful you're willing to keep trying to tell me what's going on"; "I was a teen a long time ago, so I need to have things explained to me that we both wish I knew." We find the courage to apologize—"I'm so sorry, please forgive me"—and then we try to fix it any way we can. We get better doing this in a *general* way; I promise you that it gets easier to admit mistakes as time goes on. Still, there is a specific strategy to learn to reattune with each adolescent. Just like the mothers in Tronick's research, we'll have to figure it out through trial and error as we go along in that *particular* intersubjective dance. You'll need to check in with your own gut about whether the rupture has been addressed. If it's still in the room for you, that means it's still in the room.

Open Spaces

It's hard to imagine a more awkward silence than the one between a therapist who has run out of questions and an adolescent who has nothing to say. But we want our clients to learn to tolerate anxiety; so sitting together in the face of this mutual discomfort can also be a kind of practice. Whether or not an adolescent is talkative, we do well simply to be curious about what might happen next for us as we sit together in those quiet spaces. Managing or covering over and filling these self-conscious moments can suggest that we don't think the adolescent can handle them. And for quieter kids, our ease in the silence holds respect and conveys, "I accept you as you are." Some adolescents are so used to fending off adult inquisitions that they are on guard before we ask our first question. We can provide a corrective relational experience by being less intrusive, perhaps clearing the way for them to come toward us.

See also if the moment of quiet offers a tacit invitation to head inward and then toward some conversation that's even richer; or whether you can cultivate a silence that's simply peaceful and connective, if only for a blink or two. I once worked with a girl for the better part of a year. After we'd gotten to know each other, we sometimes sat in amiable quiet for a few minutes here and there as she made watercolor paintings or just lounged on the couch. One memorable winter day, cozy under a blanket, she stretched and sighed loudly before saying to me contentedly, "You know, Marti, this is the only place I can just be me with someone else." Foolishly, I'd been a little worried that I should be doing more than simply sitting there beaming at her (somewhat approximating the way parents have gazed at their infants since the beginning of time).

Truthfully, though, for many of us, including me, it's really hard work staying present without the distraction of conversation or an activity to do. Many of us have the discerning editorial voice in our heads that booms, "What are you going to write about *this* session? What will your supervisor say when she hears this silent tape? You're getting paid to pay careful attention to a kid daydreaming under a blanket? And the objectives of this hour are what, exactly?"

We have to make plenty of room for the right brain to show up. It's worth it because, as you'll come to see, affect and unconscious material tend to be quite responsive to silence. Talking can let us into an adolescent's world, of course, but it can also keep us far, far away.

Stay Connected

In this work, we are paying attention moment-to-moment to any infor-mation that might facilitate or repair connection. We are working to be as aware as we can of all the unconscious (and conscious) information transmitted in the experience of being together—between our bodies in a glance, a gesture, a slight alteration of posture or facial expression, revealed so fleetingly that we may not be sure we caught it. And we're likely to flat-out miss those micro-moments of attunement if we're just paying attention to verbal content. Luckily for therapy, we'll usually get quite a few opportunities to make adjustments, even within the single hour, when we start noticing more carefully.

But you'll know it when it happens: shifts in empathy and attun-ement alter connection in an instant, and can define a session more than all the processing of the other 49 minutes. The knowing grab of the eye, a shared chuckle, the turning toward or away, the change in breathing, focus, or level of activity: we can take note of it all, commenting or questioning just now and then—when we can say it with curiosity, and without judgment or shaming.

I love Marotto's (2003) felicitous expression, *unflinching empathy*, and believe that concept is essential to sustaining this relationship with traumatized teens. Such empathic responding helps us pay attention to moments when our clients' arousal is overwhelming, or when they are feeling too vulnerable and begin to dissociate. We empathically make room and give language to some of the feelings that they have warded off as too dangerous or dysregulating to experience on their own. We try not to flinch even when we may have alternative, more compelling adult narratives, informed skepticism, or our own feelings about their feelings.

Notably, also, we don't have to attend in some special way just to distressed or negative emotions. In fact, for many of these adolescents, the novelty of happiness, pride, gratitude, delight, or even simple con-nection can be as destabilizing and anxiety provoking as the bad feel-ings. When strong attachment-based feelings have become associated with traumatic loss, the good ones become a threat, too.

Offer simple reflections about what you notice or about what might be happening in their bodies. Try to avoid asking too many questions, especially if you can figure out how to make a curious, empathic obser-vation instead. Open-ended questions that work well with adults can feel disconnecting and invasive to a traumatized teen. By contrast, a tenta-tive, empathic response can keep them close, help to co-regulate, and give them the words they don't necessarily have to label their complex emotional experiences. We reflect back:

"That was really scary."

"She's being so unfair, and you're *mad*!"

"Oh, you're holding yourself so tightly today."

"That's painful, not knowing who is on your team."

"So lonely . . . "

"Part of you really hates him."

"So you just can't count on her when you need her."

"I'm guessing you'd feel sort of resentful or let down."

"I think a lot of kids in this situation would be pretty mad or frustrated too."

"Oh, that sounds so wonderful, I think my heart might be singing if that happened to me!"

If you want to ask about specific feelings, you can do it more connectively by emphasizing you're just wondering: "Maybe you feel . . . a little sad about this?" Or ask it in such a way that you're inviting both affect and naming (getting the whole brain into the act): "Of all the things that worry you, what worries you the most right now?" In any event, try to keep your stance a little curious and tentative—no one likes to be told how she feels, probably least of all a traumatized adolescent. Keep guessing, offer some possibilities, and prepare to be wrong. It's been my experience that some adolescents say I am clueless when I'm spot on; others have no idea how they feel, or what the word is to describe it, and benefit from the labeling itself. And best of all, when I've guessed and mirrored the experience just so, through words and tone, so it resonates deeply, the adolescent gets to *feel felt*.

Be the Adult

The therapeutic relationship here is both real and transferential. Thus when we work with traumatized adolescents, we need to make sense of who we are to the teen both as our authentic adult selves, and as stand-ins for all the other adults they have ever known or needed. And it can feel especially complicated because we quite literally may engage in "reparenting" relationships with these adolescents—although we clearly know that we are not their parents. We try to appreciate how the adolescent client views us on these multiple levels and to step up willingly and intentionally as the *only grown-up in the room*, if not in their whole intimate lives.

Devaluing our importance to them as caring adults might be humble or efficient, or fit theoretically into more manualized paradigms that "anyone could do." It might somehow get us off the hook, write off a therapy that is less effective than we wanted, or say goodbye without pain, and forget them more easily. Still, that stance really reflects a kind of "childism"; we can too readily reduce ourselves to the role of technician, or interventionist, and keep the work from getting "too personal." But these teens are not going to get generically healthier; they are going to become more like us. They will learn about love, repair, problem solving, and what regulation feels like from how we do these things—from how we live in the world, and from being in this specific, unique relationship (Lewis, Amini, & Lannon, 2001).

And so sometimes it makes no sense to be neutral with the same equanimity with which we're trained to treat adults. Yes, our adolescent clients are sharing deeply personal information with us, and we know how fast we lose contact when we start judging and preaching. But they are also telling us about their lives because they want us to care. We have an obligation of sorts to share our experience of being with them—from the unique vantage point of perceiving them with our adult senses.

We might want to say, for example:

"I'm feeling really worried about you right now because you're not being safe."
"This is frustrating for both of us. I wonder what we could each do to make it better."
"I'm very proud of you. Did you know that?"
"I'm a little anxious about telling you the answer is 'no' because I imagine you'll be very disappointed."
"If I were in your shoes, I'd be confused, too."
"It's been a long time since I was your age, but I wonder if my experience with bullying might be helpful."
"It's your choice, and I wasn't invited to that party, so I won't be there, but can I tell you what I think might happen if you go?"
"I'll love you just the same whatever you decide, but I wonder if I might get half a vote on what you might say to your teacher?"
"Of course, it's true as you say, that the world is really different than back when I was 16, but one thing that never changes is how much a broken heart can hurt."
"I remember what happened the last time you had this fight with your mom, so I wonder if I could make a prediction here?"
"I know it feels terrible now, but I can promise you it will get better."
"You are one of the bravest kids I've ever met."

Be Kind

Sometimes when I supervise graduate students, I see them getting tangled in theory and in their own heartfelt desire to say or do the correct, healing thing. These neocortical distractions pull them up into their own heads and out of relationship. I hear these promising young trainees adopt an officious, helpful tone, or the deliberate mannerisms of someone trying to sound like a grown-up or, worse, a therapist. They might offer bountiful psychoeducation and interpretation, or ask for information that gets them deep into the weeds of a narrative, to keep the conversation going. None of this is particularly harmful, of course, but I want them to get out of their minds and back into connection when they find themselves overthinking this way. I suggest to them, "If you don't know what to say or do, just be kind. You can even ask yourself, 'What would I say to a friend here?' "

Therapists working with high-risk teens are under a lot of pressure to do something transformative in every session, to fix what seems broken in the room, to make it better fast. Sometimes this desire stems from expectations of supervisors or insurance companies, or compassion for desperate parents or frighteningly dysregulated clients. Before we try to do anything else, though, we need to frontload empathy and validation; indeed, empathy and validation may be all that are needed in this moment. *It never hurts to be kind.* And no matter what we do next, first we must make the limbic connection that lets our adolescent clients know that we get how hard this is for them, and that we're respectful of that. If it were easy to fix, they would have done that already. So if you don't know what to do, listen fully—allow yourself to feel for and with them. Be kind. For these kids, *that's* an intervention.

Keep Guessing about Emotions

When treating traumatized teens, try—to the extent it is possible for a therapist—*not* to ask them anything along the lines of, "How did you feel about that?" You may already have discovered, perhaps even repeatedly, that this is generally a dead-end line of inquiry, and I encourage you to give it up. Of course, it's really helpful to be able apply a label to an affect, and from time to time, you may encounter adolescents who have an accurate and nuanced vocabulary for their internal experience. But don't expect such insight, or be disappointed or frustrated when the response you get is a blank stare, or "Fine," or "I don't know."

Indeed, it's best to assume that for a while you'll be the one doing *all* of that emotion-naming work. In most situations, it's more effective simply to guess and wonder about feelings, even if you aren't so sure yourself, or are pretty clueless about what's going on. Offer a few ideas and be prepared to be wrong: "You seem kind of worried, or maybe angry; is that right?"

Name the cues that you're picking up on that led you to make that guess: "Okay, maybe you're not mad, but you're raising your voice, so that's why I wondered if you were." You might also normalize the feelings so you convey acceptance, and stay away from shaming: "I hear you tell me you don't feel mad, but I can understand how someone would be mad if they didn't think people were listening." You could also simply help by generalizing. You'll keep the naming in the room but deflect it from being directed at them: "A lot of kids I know would feel mad in this situation." Or, as I discussed above, you can always use your own adult experience in the service of the therapy: "I think if this happened to me, I'd be pretty angry." Remember, the goal is to listen, observe, be curious, and guess as compassionately as you can. Try to help your clients be in a conversation about their emotional experiences even when they don't yet have the vocabulary themselves.

And traumatized teens are often so disconnected from their inner worlds that they may not even know they are feeling anything. I've seen clients get teary and flushed, grin impishly, shake their feet, and clench their fists without even knowing they are upset, amused, agitated, or furious. We guess from our experience of them and what we see, and maybe invite them to try to help us put their body language into words. Even if they deny all of it and can't make the leap, they still get exposed to our concern and curiosity. Developing a shared emotional language makes hard feelings less isolating and scary. As PBS television host Mr. Rogers once so succinctly stated: "If it's mentionable, it's manageable."

Talk about Small Details

Adolescents live in the small details of their lives. We do well, then, to join them and invite greater depth and meaning into those seemingly superficial conversations about being dissed in the lunchroom, the rude DMV lady, or the nagging mother. By encouraging teens to share real moments from the day so they are practically relived in the therapy room, we further help them to develop a coherent identity narrative. Our affective engagement and curiosity help them understand and integrate events that follow in a connected sequence and, in real time, to be aware of feelings that might have been part of the original experience.

See what happens when you stop trying to "do deep trauma work" and explore actual current events in as much detail as the teen can handle. There is meaning everywhere, even standing in line at the DMV or arguing with the principal. We get so confused by content and whose agenda we need to serve in a given hour. My advice is usually to go with the flow; don't be worried if you are "just" talking about another fight at school. If that's what's most readily available, see what happens when you go all the way in, with your heart and mind fully engaged.

Help your adolescent client collect and connect the dots formed by seemingly superficial data points. Be curious. Lean forward and ask what people were wearing, where they sat, what happened first, who else was there? Find out what happened before, and next, and try to bring affect along. Say, for example, "You told him *that*? Wow. What did he do when he heard it?" Stay involved with both physical and verbal attunement. Let her story get to you so you can share in authentic feeling: "That's so funny!" "No way!" "That DMV lady didn't know who she was dealing with!" Ask for a demonstration if the story has some elements of physicality in it: "Show me how you walked away instead of fighting." "Act out for me how she wagged her finger in your face." "Can you do both parts?" "Can I take the part of the DMV lady so I can really feel what it must have been like in that interaction?" Keep eliciting details until there aren't any more. Don't change the subject until the story is told as richly and completely as possible.

When an adolescent client makes a general statement, press a bit for a specific example. If she claims that no one at school likes her, ask about a particular event that proves this to her, and, with great compassion, go as deep as she'll let you into the details of what happened in that one instance: "He just moved to a different chair when you sat down? Oh, no! Then what happened?" Every specific story you get to hear brings you closer to the adolescent's internal working model of relationships and her emotional world, and gives you a better chance to recognize these patterns in your relationship, too.

Have Fun

Trauma therapy is, much too often, serious business. When we think about "doing trauma work," we may assume, incorrectly, that it shouldn't be fun or playful. Remember, these are not adults we are dealing with, and our young clients probably didn't get much time to "just be kids" before they hit adolescence, making them less resilient now. Neglect and abuse interfere not only with secure attachment, but also with the behavioral system of exploration and play. Without a secure base, the capacity to play gets compromised; traumatized teens can't manage the wide range of arousal states or the level of undefended absorption that play requires. The unpredictability and novelty of fun may be too evocative of the unpredictability and danger of earlier traumatic experiences. In addition, our adolescent clients don't play perhaps because they may have come to associate positive affect with vulnerability to ridicule, disapproval, disdain, or even violence. All affective states have their perils for these adolescents, including—or even especially—the ones that we might associate with a good time.

So in this therapy, we don't just pay attention to the trauma story and attachment-related problems, but we're on the alert for opportunities to engage more joyfully, too. These may be just micro "now moments" where eyes meet and knowing smiles are exchanged, or offer the possibility for more expansive, fun times. Linger on a chuckle, laugh at yourself (but never at the teen, unless you are laughing together and he clearly gets his own joke); expand on something that seems ironic, comical, or mildly amusing. Notice when the connection feels lighter, or something tough has been accomplished; a little relief is also worth registering. As much as tears, laughter can be an attachment-based affect (e.g., Nelson, 2008), so it can be healing therapy to share joy, too.

We want our traumatized clients to develop a much broader platform on which to build their emotional hardiness. The window of affect tolerance needs to be wide enough to also accommodate pleasure and spontaneity. As Allan Schore (2003) writes, "Affect regulation is not just the reduction of affective intensity, the dampening of negative emotion. It also involves an amplification, an intensification of positive emotion, a condition necessary for more complex self organization" (p. 78). Therapy with traumatized adolescents can be really tough, sad, wrenching work, but it needs to be more than that, so they can live fuller, happier, more integrated lives when we're done.

CONCLUDING THOUGHTS

All emotional expression is attachment based. Whatever these teens reveal or hide, and whatever wells up in us when we're with them, is ultimately the most important information we have to work with. The process of treatment, then, helps adolescents safely bring a broader range of expressiveness into therapy, especially those really big feelings that show up as the many variations of joy, sorrow, terror, and rage. In real time, we step up to co-regulate, helping them feel—and then feel better. Traumatized teens tend to have a very narrow bandwidth of expressiveness. Living with hypervigilance and a fiery nervous system, they often teeter all day long on the brink of dysregulation. Tiny provocations can send them over the edge. A wider range of emotional expression gives them a much larger and sturdier platform for living in the world.

Over time, this approach has a secondary, but equally important effect: it builds courage in highly anxious adolescents. Along with all their worries, these teens also contend repeatedly with cause for *discouragement*. For example, Louisa struggled to make it through a day at school without getting a migraine, or starting a fight, or retreating into a dissociative fog. And like Louisa, most of the adolescents we work with need to become grittier, better insulated, and more resilient if they are to suffer less. The compassionate relationship is fundamentally fortifying; it provides the *en*couragement they'll need to face inevitable experiences of helplessness, failure, and rejection. Secure love heals attachment trauma. When we bring our best, most mindful, and heartful selves to the therapy relationship, our adolescent clients can truly feel they are not alone anymore.

FIVE RECOMMENDED PRACTICES

1. Foster an effective dependence so the adolescent can learn that you are reliable and kind, and that she is worthy of care and concern. Make promises you can keep; create routines that are special for this relationship.

2. Talk about what is happening right here and now in the room to help make connections between what they've experienced in other relationships and so assume will happen in this therapy relationship. Provide actual corrective relational experiences that ensure this one is different and better.

3. Take full adult responsibility for what happens in treatment, including repairing ruptures, guessing and naming feelings (instead of asking about feelings), and staying emotionally present and regulated. You are the adult and this therapy is up to you.

4. Have deep, wide-ranging, "nontherapeutic" discussions about whatever incidental and trivial topics may be of interest; ask animated engaged, specific questions, and delve as deeply as possible into whatever is on a teen's mind. Adolescents live in the small details of their lives and you will find meaning when you can join them exploring all the nooks and crannies.

5. Expand the emotional platform for traumatized teens, attending to the broadest possible range of emotions, opening further their window of tolerance for all kinds of affect. Find and notice occasions for laughter and pleasure, too. Remember that having fun can be even harder for some of your anxious, hypervigilant clients, and they will get stronger and more regulated when they are able to *enjoy* being with you.

REFERENCES

Johnson, S. (2009). Attachment theory and emotionally focused therapy for individuals and couples. In J. Obegi & E. Berant (Eds.), *Attachment theory and research in clinical work with adults* (pp. 410–433). New York: Guilford Press.

Jordan, J. V. (2010). *Relational-cultural therapy*. Washington, DC: American Psychological Association.

Lewis, T., Amini, F., & Lannon, R. (2001). *A general theory of love*. New York: Random House.

Marotto, S. (2003). Unflinching empathy: Counselors and tortured refugees. *Journal of Counseling and Development, 81*, 111–114.

Nelson, J. (2008). Laugh and the world laughs with you: An attachment perspective on the meaning of laughter in psychotherapy. *Clinical Social Work Journal, 36*, 41–49.

Schore, A. (2003). *Affect regulation and the repair of the self*. New York: Norton.

Siegel, D. (2012). *Pocket guide to interpersonal neurobiology: An integrative handbook of the mind*. New York: Norton.

Tronick, E. Z. (2007). *The neurobehavioral and social-emotional development of infants and children*. New York: Norton.

Silencing and the Culture of Sexual Violence

The "Shadow Abuser"

Sarah Caprioli
David A. Crenshaw

Secrets can be heavy burdens to carry. What they lack in physical form they make up for in weight, and while this may seem an unlikely arrangement according to our understanding of the physical universe, most of us know all too well the psychological heaviness of secrecy. Secrets create shadows—dark spots on the soul that isolate, shame, and silence those who carry them. For children carrying secrets of sexual abuse, the silence can be deafening and the load especially burdensome. This kind of abuse forces children to experience and respond to their victimization in silence (Caprioli & Crenshaw, 2015), but their voices are further suppressed by their very existence in the modern world. This is because we have created a society that values toxic and violent views of sexuality, which adds a thick layer of shame and silence to an already voiceless population. What is it like for child victims of sexual abuse growing up in a culture that normalizes and promotes sexual violence? For many, the experience can feel oddly familiar. Interaction with their environment at every turn exposes children to the toxic effects of living in a culture of sexual violence, and further victimizes them. When children begin to feel the impact of victimization by the very culture they live in, they have had their first metaphorical encounter with the "shadow abuser."

The concept of a culture of sexual violence has its origins in early 1970s feminist theory, which described the intentional linking of sexuality and violence in modern Western society (Herman, 1984). The term "rape culture" was coined around this time to refer to the complex set of beliefs and behaviors that normalize and encourage sexual aggression of men toward women. In a rape culture, sexual violence is seen as a normal, inevitable, and even desirable part of life (Buchwald, Fletcher, & Roth, 1993). Expanding on this idea, a culture of sexual violence is one in which violence and sex are intertwined to such an extent as to make it virtually impossible to separate one from the other. It is a society that promotes the hypersexualization of just about everything: children, adults, products and services, and even the most mundane experiences and interactions. The culture of sexual violence identifies aggression and dominance as core traits of masculinity and justifies the perpetration of sexual violence in all its forms, from microaggressions and harassment to sexual assault and rape. Although children and adults alike are affected by life in a culture of sexual violence, the experience of children who have also been sexually abused may be qualitatively different. For child victims of sexual abuse, the culture of sexual violence can feel like a living, breathing entity; a kind of "shadow abuser" that behaves and affects them in ways that mimic those abusers who take human form. The culture both grooms them and coerces them into silence. It creates shame about their bodies and their worth. It whispers to them that they deserved what happened to them and destroys their credibility with the people who might otherwise have helped them. The culture of sexual violence works in tandem with sexual aggressors, and in fact one would not be able to survive without the other. Anti-pornography researcher and activist Gail Dines (2010) provides a chilling illustration of this phenomenon in her book, *Pornland: How Porn Has Hijacked Our Sexuality,* where she recalls an interview with a child rapist in a Connecticut state prison. When asked how he prepared his victim for abuse, the offender casually replied that he actually never had to do much, because the culture did so much of the grooming for him.

In this chapter, we explore the silencing of child victims of sexual abuse within the context of a culture of sexual violence. We contend that the experience of growing up in a sociocultural environment that promotes toxic views of sexuality creates vulnerabilities to sexual violence and reinforces silence in child victims. We describe how this process of silencing may manifest in the therapy room, as well as the complex and multilayered role clinicians must be willing to take in order to root out the insidious impact of this cultural phenomenon and help children to reclaim their stolen voices.

SOCIAL AND CULTURAL TOXICITY

For more than two decades, James Garbarino (1995) has been writing about raising children in a socially toxic environment. Garbarino has focused on such social toxins as poverty, violence, especially the proliferation of guns, economic pressures on families, disrupted family relationships, the trauma of terrorism, and the pervasive fear many children experience, not just our children and youth growing up in what Garbarino refers to as the "war zones" of the inner cities. Garbarino sees these social toxins as akin to the poisons in our environment such as air pollution, PCBs in water, and pesticides in food. We would add to that list of social toxins the sexualization of our children, even our young children. In more recent writing on social toxicity, Garbarino (2011) cited the evolution of media technology since television was introduced in most homes in the 1950s. Digital video recordings over ubiquitous smartphones ensure that whatever images are toxic for both adults and children to see will come to life on TV, computer, tablet, or phone screens in nearly every home in America. We would also add to the toxic social context attitudes and myths supporting *rape culture* and *hypermasculinity*, which we view as *toxic masculinity*.

THE SILENT SCREAM

Imagine falling into an abandoned well. Picture in your mind and try to feel in your body what it might feel like if you screamed as loud as you can and no one heard you. After a while, the futility of screaming at the top of your lungs would give way to exhaustion and a weary resignation resulting in silence. The screams no longer come because there is no one who can hear them, but inside they continue in silent desperation. This is the best that we can do to try to capture through imagery the experience of a child not heard and eventually unable to call out (silenced) because those who would be expected to help don't hear the muffled sounds coming from the dark reaches (culture of sexual violence) of the well.

The depth of the well signifies how early the inappropriate sexualization of young children begins. How often have we seen loving, well-intended parents or grandparents refuse to teach children the correct terms for their body parts and instead insist on using "cutesy" language to refer to genitalia? Although this may seem a harmless substitution, the practice of nicknaming children's private parts sends a strong message that these parts are somehow different and cannot be talked about openly. Worse still, children at times are admonished for using accurate terminology, as if they had said a "dirty" word. Over time, children begin to associate the very idea of sexuality with silence and shame. Most parents and grandparents would be highly disturbed to learn that they had contributed to laying the groundwork for rape culture, but that is exactly the reason we wish to delineate this subtle and insidious process and bring it to the awareness of child therapists and, by extension, to the awareness of the general public.

What well-meaning child therapist has not said to a little girl who shows up to a session in a pretty dress and with a bow in her hair, "Oh, you look so cute today!" On the surface it seems harmless. But what if those comments are repeated constantly not just by therapists, but teachers, coaches, parents, and grandparents? What is the unintended message here? The message to the little girl is that it is her appearance, looks, and dress that elicit attention and approval from the important adults in her life. It is because of her "cuteness" that she gains the approval of attachment and authority figures. Do we want our little girls to learn that approval hinges on their physical appearance? Boys can be exposed to this unwitting form of shaping their self-esteem as well: "My, don't you look handsome today!" "Little man, you are looking good, you are going to have the beat the girls off with a stick!" The little boy or girl may be intelligent, artistic, creative, kind, sensitive, curious, athletic, and personable, but only their physical appearance draws our attention and praise. Child therapists have become more aware and attuned to *microaggressions* (Sue, 2010) that occur in therapy as well as in everyday life all too frequently. Microaggressions, as Sue (2010) explains, are about everyday prejudice, bias, and discrimination on marginalized groups in our society, including children, that have damaging consequences. These microaggressions are potent partly because they are invisible to the perpetrators, who remain blindly unaware of the damage they are inflicting. Since they are subconscious, they can persist for long periods, in some cases throughout the child's developmental, formative years, which then can easily lead to the internalization of such microaggressions by the victim. The little girls or boys who were most frequently praised and complimented because of appearance may internalize such appraisals and view themselves as having value contingent on their physical appearance. The realization that therapists, teachers, coaches, parents, and grandparents actively foster such narrow and limited self-attitudes evokes sadness for the children but also for the well-intended adults.

WHY DO ONLY 10% OF SEXUALLY ABUSED CHILDREN DISCLOSE DURING CHILDHOOD?

You may be as startled as we were that only 10% of adults who acknowledge sexual abuse as a child disclosed during childhood (see Lyon, 2014, for a review). The culture has created a concealing and silencing force that leads 90% of child sexual abuse victims interviewed as adults to remain silent throughout their growing-up years. The *silent scream* is their constant companion during childhood and adolescence, and tragically for some, their lifelong companion.

There are multiple contributors to the silencing of children. Gaskill and Perry (Chapter 3, this volume) explain in depth the developmental limitations on cognitive and language functioning that make it hard particularly for children under the age of 12 to talk about their feelings or to fully grasp or articulate the bad things that happen to them, but in this chapter we focus primarily on the contributions of toxic cultural influences like rape culture and toxic masculinity in the silencing of children.

RAPE CULTURE

A key component of the broader culture of sexual violence in which we live is the concept of rape culture, which more specifically describes male sexual aggression toward women and women's experience of this. Although the impact of rape culture has been most widely studied in connection to the alarming rates of sexual violence on college campuses, its influence is pervasive and infiltrates almost every aspect of life in contemporary Western society. At its core, rape culture consists of beliefs, myths, and practices around gender and sexuality that normalize and even justify sexual violence. These ideas are shared and perpetuated in a number of ways, most notably by media and popular culture, politics and legislation, social systems, and direct communication between individuals and groups.

While there exists a staggering number of commonly held and harmful beliefs about gender and sexuality in contemporary Western culture, several stand out as being particularly toxic in their ability to normalize sexual violence. The idea that women and children do not own their bodies is one such belief. As described earlier in this chapter, the internalization of this belief begins early in childhood and is reinforced at every stage of life. From the time they are toddlers, children are expected to acquiesce to requests for physical affection from adults in the form of hugs, kisses, and other types of physical touch. In many cases, resistance to such demands results in the child's being chastised or punished for her "disobedience." From the start, children are taught that their bodies are not their own, and that decisions about what happens to their bodies are made independently of their own level of comfort or consent. As children grow and start to explore their environments, this idea is reinforced over and over again. "Street harassment" is a term commonly used to refer to the practice of making unsolicited and sexualized comments, jokes, expressions, and gestures to individuals in public places. Overwhelmingly perpetrated by males against females, this type of uninvited attention is often aggressive and objectifying. The message inherent in such behavior is that when women's bodies occupy public spaces, they are fair game for scrutiny and displays of male sexual aggression and dominance. Here again we see a powerful manifestation of the belief that women do not own their bodies in that they have no choice regarding their exposure to such scrutiny and indeed are often further victimized if they protest or respond negatively to this behavior. Recently, the anti-street harassment organization Hollaback! in partnership with Cornell University released the results of the largest international street harassment survey to date (Livingston, 2015). The study surveyed 16,607 participants in 22 countries about their experiences of street harassment. Relevant to this discussion is the finding regarding participants' age during their first experience of harassment. Globally, the majority of women reported first instances of street harassment during puberty, and 85% of U.S. women reported being harassed before the age of 17. Even more disturbingly, approximately 67% of women in the United States reported that their first experience of street harassment occurred before age 14. The study suggests that, as girls develop, they are regularly exposed to messages that their bodies are public property and that others have innate rights to those bodies. The shadow abuser is at work, exposing their insecurities and eroding their sense of autonomy even as they walk to school or play outside.

Cultural messages that women lack ownership of their own bodies are not only perpetuated by individuals who internalize and act on these beliefs, but also by entire systems that create laws and legislation based on stereotypes around gender and sexuality. One particularly egregious example of this is the issue of spousal rape. The United States justice system has long been reluctant to get involved in issues deemed "domestic matters" and until recently did not even recognize spousal rape as a crime. The belief, which is still held today by many law enforcement and criminal justice professionals among others, is that it is impossible for a man to rape his wife because sex is a duty that wives are expected to fulfill. In fact, it was not until 1993 that spousal rape was made illegal in at least one section of the sexual offense codes in all 50 states (Bennice

& Resick, 2003). Even today, many states persist in qualifying spousal rape as a crime only if certain conditions are met. For example, in Alabama, spousal rape must include the *overt* use of force or threat of force in order for the crime to be prosecuted. Unofficially, these crimes are still widely viewed with skepticism and not taken seriously due to the widespread belief that this type of crime is not "real" rape (Bennice & Resick, 2003).

Another foundational belief typically present in a rape culture is the concept of woman-as-seductress (Herman, 1984). According to this belief, women and girls possess almost magical powers that cause men to be rendered helpless to control their impulses. Women are seen essentially as sexual objects who are constantly "asking for it" in the ways they dress, behave, and generally exist. The application of the woman-as-seductress belief most often results in victim blaming, where blame is transferred from the perpetrator to the victim, thereby making the victim responsible for her own victimization (Caprioli & Crenshaw, 2015). Examples of this abound in the media and popular culture, where women are often depicted in hypersexualized ways that leave men "no choice" but to pursue them in a sexually aggressive manner. One need only turn on the television, go online, read a magazine, or walk into almost any retail store to be bombarded by imagery rife with examples of the seductress archetype. Children viewing these images may hear the shadow abuser murmuring to them, whispering that this is the beginning and end of their value as humans. The idea of woman as seductress is also readily seen in daily life. Sexual assault victims commonly report being questioned by family, friends, and law enforcement about what they were wearing, how much they had to drink, and whether they may have "led him on." In addition, adding insult to injury, there is evidence that adolescent rape victims are viewed with greater skepticism by juries than younger victims (Bottoms & Goodman, 1994).

The belief that women possess sexual power over men is not limited to adult females, but also extends to adolescents and even young children. One alarming example of this concept applied to children can be illustrated by the first author's work with "Jane," an adult woman who was sexually abused as a child. Jane's stepfather began abusing her at age 9, and the abuse continued daily for about 5 years until age 14, when Jane was finally able to summon the courage to tell her mother. Upon hearing her disclosure, Jane's mom called her stepfather into the room to confront him directly on the accusation. Jane's stepfather admitted that they had indeed been engaged in a long-term sexual relationship, but only because Jane had "seduced" him (at age 9!) and coerced him into it. Incredibly, Jane's mom accepted this explanation, noting that Jane was a "slutty" child, and forced Jane to apologize for her promiscuous behavior. The crime was never reported, and Jane's mom and stepfather remain married today.

SEXUAL VIOLENCE MYTHS

A byproduct of the perpetuation of faulty beliefs regarding gender and sexuality is the widespread cultural acceptance of sexual violence myths. Sexual violence myths begin with stereotypes about sexuality that are then applied to the actual practice of sexual assault. We encounter these myths almost everywhere, from film, television, advertising, and other forms of media to our criminal justice and mental health systems. The fact that they are false makes almost no difference in how frequently they are referenced and used to shame and silence victims of sexual assault, and in fact they seem almost impervious to attack. A quick sampling of popular culture reveals a bevy of myths about sexual violence: most sexual assaults are perpetrated by strangers; the majority of reports of sexual violence are false; rape is a crime of passion; and there is a "right" way to react as a victim just to name a few (Buchwald et al., 1993; Lonsway, Archambault, & Lisak, 2009). Although all of the myths discussed here have been unequivocally debunked (Berzofsky, Krebs, Langton, Planty, & Smiley-McDonald, 2013; Lonsway et al., 2009) they persist in informing our collective understanding of sexual violence and serve to qualify individual experiences of sexual aggression. For women and girls growing up in this culture, the message is clear: victims of sexual violence who come forward will be met with scrutiny, skepticism, and often with outright disbelief. Victims encounter this reaction not only from their friends and family, but also from the many professionals with whom they must interact in order to pursue justice and begin to heal from these crimes. The power of these myths to influence how sexually violent crimes are investigated and prosecuted can be illustrated by my (SC) work with a Sexual Assault Nurse Examination (SANE) program, in which a SANE nurse reported disturbing conduct by a police officer sent to the hospital to interview a victim. Upon his arrival, the SANE nurse told the officer that the adolescent victim had disclosed sexual assault by an acquaintance and was interested in filing a police report. Before hearing any details of the case, the officer informed the nurse that he had a foolproof method of determining whether alleged victims were telling the truth. The officer stated that the first question he asks is whether the victim experienced an orgasm, since achieving orgasm would obviously mean that the sex was consensual. Victim advocates on the case were appropriately appalled, but the officer's superiors did not see any need for disciplinary action or retraining despite extensive advocacy. Survivors of sexual assault routinely feel the piercing gaze of the shadow abuser poring over every aspect of their story (and perhaps their bodies), and twisting their words into a new narrative in which even young victims may be painted as attention-seeking liars.

HYPERSEXUALIZATION OF YOUNG GIRLS

Perhaps one of the most disturbing illustrations of rape culture is the large-scale hypersexualization of young girls in Western society. While this phenomenon has been well documented in the academic literature (American Psychological Association Task Force on the Sexualization of Girls, 2007; Caprioli & Crenshaw, 2015; Tishelman & Geffner, 2010), the evidence in everyday life is overwhelming. Music, television, toys, games, and clothing are just some of the places girls encounter both explicit and implicit messages that their worth is intrinsically tied to their sexuality. Retailers market soft pink purses filled with plush lipstick and blush to babies, excitedly proclaiming to parents that their 6-month-old baby can now be "just like mommy!" A trip to almost any department store turns up cropped tops, bikinis, and high heels before one even gets out of the toddler section (Goodin, Van Denburg, Murnen, & Smolak, 2011). What do girls do with these messages? The term "self-sexualization" refers to the process of internalizing sexualized messages gleaned from the larger culture (Starr & Ferguson, 2012). Girls exposed to sexualizing images, products, and attitudes tend to incorporate these stereotyped gender roles into their own identities over time and to emulate others who embody these ideals. Alarmingly, this process can be seen even with young children. Starr and Ferguson (2012) demonstrated just how strong the pull of cultural influences can be by using paper dolls to illustrate self-sexualization in girls age 6 to 9. The girls were asked to choose between two dolls: one dressed in very tight and revealing "sexy" clothes, and the other in a trendy but loose and nonrevealing outfit. Participants overwhelmingly chose the "sexy" doll when asked which doll they would want to look like, and additionally believed that the sexy doll was more popular than her covered-up friend.

The hypersexualization of young girls is incredibly difficult to combat in part because of the success of mainstream culture in idealizing the sexualized female form. Girls *want* to look this way and readily adopt appearances and behaviors that mimic the images they are exposed to. It is perhaps the most insidious type of indoctrination into rape culture because it is hungrily looked for and eagerly absorbed by its victims. The shadow abuser is ever present, gently grooming and guiding those children with unmet needs for approval and acceptance until they are willing participants in their own victimization.

TOXIC MASCULINITY

Toxic masculinity refers to the need to dominate, aggressively compete, devalue women, and to engage in homophobia and sometimes wanton violence in order for males in the culture to feel manly (Kupers, 2005). The prison setting in which Kupers based his study tends to intensify toxic masculinity. Kupers clearly states that there are exceptions to every characterization of masculinity, and toxic masculinity does not apply to all males, even in prison settings. The Australian researcher Connell (1987) coined the term *hegemonic masculinity* to refer to the dominant view of masculinity in a particular historical context. In contemporary American and European cultures, Connell observed that two main features stand out: domination of women and a hierarchy of intermale dominance (Kupers, 2005). Other features include ruthless competitiveness, inability to express emotion other than anger, denial of weakness or dependence, and anxiety about the views of others for any deviations from the hegemonic norm—the fear that they will not be considered "real men" (Kupers, 2005).

   Toxic masculinity can influence adolescent males to engage in robberies or violent acts to prove their toughness and manliness to gain admission to gangs. In addition, they may view date rape or joining in a gang rape as a badge proving their masculinity. Punitive environments such as supermaximun prisons tend to incite and worsen the problems associated with toxic masculinity (Kupers, 2005). Since the domination of women is intrinsic to the prevailing cultural view of masculinity, toxic masculinity is destructive not only to women but also to men. Hypermasculinity severely limits men in reaching their full potential for intimate and satisfying relationships with others.

THE IMPACT OF TOXIC MASCULINITY
ON CHILDREN AND FAMILIES

Hypermasculinity is detrimental to children. If domination and devaluation of women are witnessed repeatedly in the interactions of their parents, and children are exposed to countless interactions within the family where power and control are dominant motivations, the result is toxic. One of the most robust impacts may be the lack of empathy. If each member of the family is determined to be right, to control and dominate, there can be no empathy (Fussner & Crenshaw, 2008). Unwittingly, the potential of the children in intimate and satisfying relationships with others will be stunted as well. In subtle but important ways, the contributing influence of the shadow abuser is growing.

In family environments where power and control drive the interactions between caregivers and between caregivers and their children, the children learn two things: they learn tactics to avoid and evade (e.g., silence), and they learn how to be controlling themselves, both of which will limit them in their social and later intimate relationships (Bonime, 1989). We believe that the vast majority of parents do the best they can to offer healthy models of intimate relationships and it has often been said that the greatest gift that parents can give to their children is a loving relationship with the other parent. What parent would set out on the conscious goal of stunting their child's growth and development? When the prevailing cultural model of what constitutes being a "real man," however, trumps this desire in the form of toxic masculinity, everyone in the family suffers. When power and control dynamics dominate family interactions, the potential for cooperation, empathy, intimacy, and satisfying relationships will be compromised and the voices of children will be silenced.

We want to point out that the foundation on which the shadow abuser builds its influence contains many planks (contributing factors) and the power/control dynamic exposed in families is only one, albeit a very important one, of many planks in that foundational floor. Cultural factors exert influence on the family, who in turn greatly influence the children raised and schooled in the family. We do not wish to point the finger of blame at any one of the planks laid down but to consider the complexity of the whole and to stimulate self-examination of all contributions to the toxic cultural influences impinging on our children's development.

INTERACTION BETWEEN CULTURAL
AND INTRAPSYCHIC DYNAMICS

Youth forced into sexual submission to meet the instinctual desires of adults suffer the trilogy of shame, stigma, and silencing (Caprioli & Crenshaw, 2015). They suffer shame and stigma paradoxically as a result of the abuse and exploitation forced on them. Van der Kolk (2015) elucidated the isolation and loneliness of trauma survivors. Who wants, is able, or is willing to hear the story of the trauma? Especially if the trauma was sexual. Consider how bizarre, how surreal the plight is of a sexual trauma survivor. Tainted by the very abuse suffered and silenced by powerful forces preventing the telling of your story of exploitation. As a result, the stigma is heightened by isolation and unbearable loneliness (the silent scream). Clearly, an important goal of treatment is overcoming the forces of silencing, stigma, secrecy, and shame to reclaim not only their voice but also their sense of self.

TREATMENT CONSIDERATIONS

For children in acute trauma states as well as those who have experienced complex and ongoing trauma, the ability to talk about their experiences may actually be compromised at the neurobiological level. Perry (2009) describes a hierarchical structure of brain function where lower neural networks in the brainstem must be well regulated in order for higher executive functions in the prefrontal cortex, such as speech, language, and memory, to operate effectively. When traumatized children encounter triggers in their environment, the brainstem can "hijack" the body, mobilizing the child's fight–flight or freeze responses in order to defend against the perceived danger (van der Kolk, 2006, 2015). This process, commonly referred to as "dysregulation," throws the child's entire system into a survival mode where basic physiological responses that foster safety are heightened while higher executive functions deemed nonessential to survival are suppressed. Energy is diverted away from the prefrontal cortex in favor of the hierarchically lower brainstem, inhibiting cognitive functions such as language and memory and subsequently the child's ability to share her story. In addition, children who have experienced complex trauma may become chronically dysregulated, as repeated abuse over time creates a patterned survival response that eventually turns into a kind of "default" setting for the child (van der Kolk, 2015).

Children who have been sexually abused may be triggered not only by reminders of the abuse, but also by their very attempts to function within a culture of sexual violence. A continuous undercurrent of sexual aggression and coercion threatens to revictimize them at any moment, preventing them from developing any long-term sense of safety. For many, the energy and resources needed just to contain the trauma in the face of so many sexually violent messages embedded in the culture can overwhelm children and keep them in a sort of perpetually dysregulated state. For these children, establishing a strong and consistent sense of safety is essential for combating silence. Safety must be created not only in the therapy environment and in the relationship with the therapist, but also within the child's body. Such efforts to "soothe" the brainstem will help to regulate the child's system and bring higher-level cognitive functioning, including language, recall, and information processing, back online. Interventions that engage the senses in a calming manner as well as the creative arts and mindfulness practices will send messages of safety to the brain, helping to ground dysregulated clients and return their bodies to their resting states (see Gaskill & Perry, Chapter 3, and Gray & Porges, Chapter 6, this volume).

Since children are effectively silenced as a result of shame, secrecy, and stigma, countering the impact of these insidious cultural influences needs to be a priority in therapy. Especially in cases of sexual abuse, the presence of this trilogy is almost universal and has been a factor in just about every case of sexual violence we have seen to date. At the root of this trilogy is the culture of sexual violence. Children are taught almost from birth that the private parts of their bodies are shameful, must be kept hidden, and are not to be talked about unless couched in "cutesy" language. At the same time, girls in particular learn from a very young age that society views their worth as being almost entirely tied to their sexuality. Is it any wonder, then, that children experience such shame and stigma when their bodies are violated in this way? Shame, secrecy, and stigma can be remarkably difficult wounds to heal, and must be addressed continuously and patiently throughout therapy. One way this trilogy may be counteracted is by soliciting stories from the children and their families that make them proud. Pursuing in both individual and/ or family sessions stories about family heroes or everyday heroes early in the therapy process can lay the groundwork for being able to talk more easily about the painful things that arouse shame. In addition, soliciting stories about times when the child was able to go against the odds and do something beyond self-expectations as well as the expectations of others is a way of expanding the theme of "everyday hero." Robert Brooks (Brooks & Goldstein, 2015) has coined the term "islands of competence" that can be found in our child clients if we aggressively pursue strengths, often hidden. The potency of the trilogy of shame, secrecy, and stigma can be dramatically lessened when the therapist focuses on strengths and resilience in the child. In addition, efforts to increase media literacy, body positivity, and self-compassion can help to inoculate the child against the constant flow of shame-inducing messages pouring out from the culture of sexual violence.

Building trust is another component essential to combatting silence, and one that simply cannot be rushed. Children growing up in the shadow of the abuser have no reason to trust a new person, regardless of the good intentions, warmth, and caring of the therapist; taking the risk of trusting the therapist can only happen after the therapist has earned such trust. In most cases, that will take considerable time and patient work. In residential settings, treating youth suffering complex trauma in my (DAC) experience, an average of 6 to 9 months is required to establish adequate trust for the child to safely unburden. It is interesting that the required time has been significantly reduced in our clinical experience by the presence of a facility dog in the sessions that significantly facilitates the building of trust. In one example, an adolescent with a horrific background was able to begin her trauma narrative through a series of letters to our facility dog within 2 weeks.

One foundational component of trust building in cases of sexual abuse is the child's belief that the other person can "hold" and handle their story. The experience of living in a culture of sexual violence has taught these children that, in many cases, their stories will be met with horror, disgust, or even disbelief. These reactions may at times be overt, but more commonly are communicated in subtle, nonverbal ways to which the child is finely attuned. The child may "test" the therapist early in the relationship by alluding to the trauma in a general way or revealing bits of the story in an attempt to see how the therapist reacts. An unintentional grimace, flinch, or sharp intake of breath can speak volumes to the sensitive ears of a silenced child. If the child feels that the therapist is not able to adequately hold this information without becoming overwhelmed, she will remain silent until she finds someone to whom she can entrust this difficult material. On the other hand, we have seen over and over again the remarkable impact that even one trustworthy and caring adult can have on the life of a traumatized child. Authentic relational engagement continues to be one of the most effective methods of buffering trauma and building resilience that we have encountered. More than any tool or technique at the therapist's disposal, the connection the therapist builds with the child will be the base on which all healing occurs.

Youth who have been sexually exploited require a depth approach to treatment. A quick fix is not feasible. Because the survivors of sexual trauma were repeatedly exposed to coercion in all of its corrosive forms—psychological, physical, social, and cultural—the attitude and actions of the therapist must not replicate coercion even in its subtler form. The therapeutic attitude should be: "I have all the time in the world for you. You need share with me only what is helpful for you to share at a time that is comfortable and safe for you." The third-party payers would run for the exits screaming, "We will not pay for it!" in all likelihood, if they were to hear such a statement. Quite unintentionally, we are sure, but the economics of mental health care have conspired against the therapeutic conditions that create a safe, comfortable context for trauma survivors to confront what has happened to them.

In today's culture of quick fixes, some will question whether there is a need to look back and confront the trauma events in order to move forward. To such doubters, Freud long ago commented that sometimes it is necessary to remember in order to forget. A noted contemporary therapist, Lesley Greenburg, best known for his contributions to emotion-focused therapy (Greenburg, 2004), wrote, "You can't leave a place until you've arrived" (p. 3). Clinical experience has repeatedly taught us that pressuring trauma clients to go further than they are prepared to go in telling their trauma story is an effective form of silencing within therapy. Perhaps no therapeutic skill is more important in trauma work than an attuned sense of timing and pacing. Paradoxically, our trauma clients have taught us that the more attention we give to safety, sensitive timing, and pacing, the quicker the work proceeds. For many years, I (DAC) have supervised other therapists in private supervision. I found therapists who were prone to have many crises and hospitalizations of clients lacked a sensitive, attuned sense of proper timing and pacing. Thus their clients experienced the therapy as unsafe. Concomitantly, these therapists were plagued with the sense of "not doing enough" in therapy and felt the need to aggressively challenge their clients in the hope for more movement and progress in the therapy. The opposite proved to be true. The more they challenged their clients, the more crises they provoked, sometimes leading to unnecessary hospitalizations. When these therapists learned to be more patient and to respect the pace that was natural and safe for their clients, the more productive the therapy became, without the interruptions of unnecessary crises and hospitalizations.

The opposite problem is also sometimes evident. We both have treated sexually abused girls and boys who had been in prior therapy where they never disclosed their abuse. These victims were unwittingly silenced by their well-meaning therapists. In every one of these instances, the youth explained that they thought they had dropped ample hints and clues of the abuse, but their therapist did not pick up on them or ask them to clarify. In work with an adolescent girl, I (DAC) vividly remember her recounting two prior separate therapy experiences, including tearing up when talking about visits with her uncle, and the therapists didn't seem to notice or ask any clarifying questions. This triggered for the girl a memory of being tucked in bed by her mother when she was 8 years old with tears rolling down her cheek, but her mother did not ask her what was upsetting her when she desperately wanted to disclose the sexual abuse by her uncle. We have learned repeatedly from our work with children and adolescents that they won't disclose to a therapist, a parent, or any other trusted adult unless they are convinced that the adult truly wants and is able to hear it. Otherwise, they will remain silent and wait for another opportunity when they hope the adult will be strong enough to hear the disclosure. If not, they will continue to protect the therapist or the parent. Sometimes it takes real courage to fully listen not only to the words said, but the words unsaid. It takes clinical courage to hear the silent scream coming from deep within the child, expressed perhaps in a single tear rolling down the cheek, or the look of sadness or fear in the eyes, or the choked-off, hesitant voice that wants to be heard. The voice, long silent, that will only be expressed and heard if we have the courage and commitment to hear what none of us, no human being, really wants to hear or believe. The story that needs to be shared of such cruelty, inhumanity, and indignities inflicted on an innocent child. We do not disparage the previous therapists who did not pick up on the cues of incipient disclosure; rather, our compassion is extended to both child and therapist because we recognize that those therapeutic conversations also took place in the presence of the "shadow abuser" that has cast darkness and has long silenced not only the child but sadly also some of the therapists who seek to help.

In order to combat the culture of sexual violence at the systemic level, therapists must be willing to fight for awareness and change within the many systems children encounter as they attempt to heal from sexual abuse. Systemic interventions require therapists to embrace advocacy as an integral part of their role, both in order to help their child clients navigate the volatile waters of their local justice, mental health, social service, and health care systems, among others, and also to begin to effect lasting change for the unknown numbers of children who have yet to pass through those systems. Most child victims of sexual abuse will never make it to this point—many will carry their secrets with them well into adulthood, and others simply will not be heard although their voices strain with the weight of their disclosure. Those who do make it will likely find themselves thrust into a series of intimidating interactions with their local justice and mental health systems, and fewer still will find the support and courage needed to successfully navigate these processes (Caprioli & Crenshaw, 2015). For child victims mired in the bureaucracy of these systems, their sense of vulnerability can be all-encompassing. Exposed and raw, they fall easy prey to the old tricks of the shadow abuser.

On their journey toward healing, children are likely to encounter the culture of sexual violence most often in the form of secondary wounding, a process by which children are further victimized by professionals and others intending to help them (Spehar, 2015). Instances of secondary wounding by professionals have been detailed throughout this chapter in the form of comments, questions, and even visceral reactions that cast shame or doubt on a child's experience. Many microaggressions are committed by helping professionals unaware of the impact of their remarks or the disapproving or judgmental facial expressions that say so much without a single word uttered. Individuals in helping roles may inadvertently pass on the toxic beliefs or behaviors characteristic of a culture of sexual violence, effectively silencing child victims even as they summon the courage over and over again to tell their stories. In addition, elements of a culture of sexual violence are in many cases woven into the very fabric of these systems, creating an institutionally sanctioned form of silencing that is not easily recognized or addressed. For example, a foundational tenet of the criminal justice process is its reliance on aggressive and adversarial questioning of witnesses at every step (Crenshaw, Stella, O'Neill-Stephens, & Walsen, 2016), which can feel eerily similar to the various forms of toxic masculinity so essential to a culture of sexual violence. Therapists who wish to combat this phenomenon must be vigilant in their role as advocates, uncovering and calling out sexually violent messages and practices wherever they threaten to silence the voices of our most vulnerable victims. They must advocate for safety and promote awareness and education among themselves and their colleagues across disciplines. Even in instances where we may not be able to help, we should never add to the wounding. Ignorance is no excuse. Sustainable systemic change that empowers rather than silences children is possible, but only through education, collaboration, and a fierce commitment to advocacy from those in the helping professions.

Not every mental health practitioner is meant to be an activist. While some of us draw energy from being on the frontlines of the battle for victims' rights, others operate most effectively behind the scenes. All of us, however, can help to effect sociocultural change. The culture of sexual violence represents the cumulative effect of myriad toxic attitudes and beliefs held first in the hearts and minds of individuals, groups, and communities. Practitioners who model awareness and growth in their own work and community settings are already helping to chip away at the underlying structure that supports the culture of sexual violence. Those professionals who do not feel the call of activism can work on a smaller scale by promoting victim-centered practices in their own work environments, bringing trainings on rape culture and toxic masculinity to their communities, or supporting community coalitions and partnerships dedicated to combatting sexual violence. Professionals who wish to take a broad approach to effecting change on a sociocultural scale may move beyond their communities to target even larger populations. We both have embraced advocacy and activism in the form of writings, presentations, and legislative action in order to advocate for nondiscriminatory treatment of women and other oppressed groups as well as protection for child witnesses in the court system. Dismantling the culture of sexual violence will take generations of dedicated and passionate work, but practitioners can choose to combat the insidious, silencing impact of this culture every day through large and small acts of awareness. In this way, we may finally begin to coax the voices of our most vulnerable clients out of the shadows of the abuser.

FIVE RECOMMENDED PRACTICES

Therapists who wish to combat the silencing impact of the culture of sexual violence must be willing not only to step outside the traditional confines of their roles, but in fact must at some point step outside of the therapy office altogether. The challenge lies in the reality that children encounter these toxic messages everywhere, and interventions that target the child in isolation do nothing to interrupt the continuous stream of misinformation to which they are exposed, creating a healing process that is fragmented at best. We contend that effective interventions not only take into account the ways in which the child has internalized and been silenced by the culture of sexual violence, but also address the people, systems, and broader cultural context that create and perpetuate these messages in the first place. In this section, we propose five levels of intervention to combat silence imposed by the culture of sexual violence: neurobiological, emotional, relational, systemic, and sociocultural.

1. Neurobiological (address dysregulation). Begin by helping the child to feel safe in his body. Understand that dysregulated children often develop hypersensitive stress response systems that compromise their ability to share and process their stories (van der Kolk, 2015). Help the child to locate, name, and describe what this feels like inside his body. Become aware of how the culture of sexual violence creates a constant undercurrent of sexual aggression and how this may intensify dysregulation. Teach the child to send messages of safety to his body by engaging his senses in a calming way. Try out different sensory-based activities like burying hands in the sand or smelling essential oils. Slow down. Understand that a deep, unrushed, felt sense of safety is a powerful antidote to silence.

2. Emotional (address shame, secrecy, and stigma). Start to pay attention to the everyday messages we receive about sex and sexuality. Practice interpreting them through a child's lens and observe how they feed the development of shame, secrecy, and stigma. Counteract this potent trilogy by cultivating resilience. Help the child develop age-appropriate media literacy, body positivity, and self-compassion. Encourage her to tell stories about family or "everyday" heroes, including the child herself. Help the child remember times when she overcame obstacles to succeed, or helped someone who was struggling.

(continued)

Look for "islands of competence" (Brooks & Goldstein, 2015) that reflect strengths the child can be proud of. Make sure she knows she is valued and valuable.

3. Relational (build trust and safety with others including the therapist). Realize that there are no shortcuts to building trust. Move slowly and with respect. Understand that traumatized children have no reason to trust new people and that you will need to show them why they should expect something different from you. Cultivate the sacred in your relationships with clients. Develop your ability to "hold" the traumatic material the child entrusts you with. Realize that the culture of sexual violence has trained them to expect others to react with horror and disgust, or not at all. Do not replicate that. Instead offer empathy, acceptance, gratitude, and know that the connection you build with the child will be the base on which all healing occurs.

4. Systemic (advocate with family, criminal justice, and mental health systems). Embrace (if you are willing and able) advocacy as an integral part of your role. Become familiar with the many systems traumatized children are expected to engage with, and learn to spot the insidious elements of rape culture and toxic masculinity woven into these systems. Watch out for secondary wounding (Spehar, 2015). Children are often silenced by well-meaning professionals unaware of the impact of their disapproving remarks or judgmental facial expressions. Be courageous in calling this out and offering empowering alternatives no matter how powerful the system you're up against. You are the voice of the silenced child. If you are too intimidated to speak, how can you ever expect the child to do the same?

5. Sociocultural (advocate and raise awareness in communities and beyond). Start small. Not every mental health practitioner is meant to be an activist, but everyone can learn to effect sociocultural change. Model awareness and growth in your own work and within your community. Chip away at the framework that supports the culture of sexual violence by promoting victim-centered practices in your own work environments or supporting local coalitions dedicated to combating sexual violence. Think big. If you have the soul of an activist, use it. Develop your expertise and share it with the world. Advocate for legislative change. Write. Present. Educate. Act.

REFERENCES

American Psychological Association Task Force on the Sexualization of Girls. (2007). Report of the APA Task Force on the Sexualization of Girls. Retrieved from *www.apa.org/pi/women/programs/girls/report-full.pdf.*

Bennice, J. A., & Resick, P. A. (2003). Marital rape: History, research, and practice. *Trauma, Violence, and Abuse, 4*(3), 228–246.

Berzofsky, M., Krebs, C., Langton, L., Planty, M., & Smiley-McDonald, H. (2013). *Female victims of sexual violence, 1994–2010.* Washington, DC: Bureau of Justice Statistics.

Bonime, W. (1989). Competitiveness and human potential. In W. Bonime (Ed.), *Collaborative psychoanalysis: Anxiety, depression, dreams, and personality change* (pp. 379–394). Rutherford, NJ: Fairleigh Dickinson University Press.

Bottoms, B. L., & Goodman, G. S. (1994). Perceptions of children's credibility in sexual assault cases. *Journal of Applied Social Psychology, 24,* 702–732.

Brooks, R. T., & Goldstein, S. (2015). The power of mindsets: Guideposts for a resilience-based treatment approach. In D. A. Crenshaw, R. T. Brooks, & S. Goldstein (Eds.), *Play therapy interventions to enhance resilience* (pp. 3–31). New York: Guilford Press.

Buchwald, E., Fletcher, P. R., & Roth, M. (1993). *Transforming a rape culture.* Minneapolis, MN: Milkweed Editions.

Caprioli, S., & Crenshaw, D. A. (2015). The culture of silencing child victims of sexual abuse: Implications for child witnesses in court. *Journal of Humanistic Psychology, 55,* 1–20.

Connell, R. W. (1987). *Gender and power.* Redwood City, CA: Stanford University Press.

Crenshaw, D. A., Stella, L., O'Neill-Stephens, E., & Walsen, C. (2016, April 14). Developmentally and trauma sensitive courtrooms. *Journal of Humanistic Psychology* (online).

Dines, G. (2010). *Pornland: How porn has hijacked our sexuality.* Boston: Beacon Press.

Fussner, A., & Crenshaw, D. A. (2008). Healing the wounds of children in a family context. In D. A. Crenshaw (Ed.), *Child and adolescent psychotherapy: Wounded spirits and healing paths* (pp. 31–48). Lanham, MD: Jason Aronson.

Garbarino, J. (1995). *Raising children in a socially toxic environment.* San Francisco: Jossey-Bass.

Garbarino, J. (2011). *The positive psychology of personal transformation: Leveraging resilience for life change.* New York: Springer.

Goodin, S. M., Van Denburg, A., Murnen, S. K., & Smolak, L. (2011). "Putting on" sexiness: A content analysis of the presence of sexualizing characteristics in girls' clothing. *Sex Roles, 65,* 1–12.

Greenburg, L. (2004). Emotion-focused therapy. *Clinical Psychology and Psychotherapy, 11,* 3–16.

Herman, D. F. (1984). The rape culture. In J. Freeman (Ed.), *Women: A feminist perspective* (pp. 45–53). Palo Alto, CA: Mayfield.

Kupers, T. A. (2005). Toxic masculinity as a barrier to mental health treatment in prison. *Journal of Clinical Psychology, 61,* 713–724.

Livingston, B. A. (2015). Hollaback! and Cornell University international street harassment survey project. Retrieved from *http://ihollaback.org/cornell-international-survey-on-street-harassment/#us.*

Lonsway, K. A., Archambault, J., & Lisak, D. (2009). False reports: Moving beyond the issue to successfully investigate and prosecute non-stranger sexual assault. *The Voice, 3*(1), 1–11.

Lyon, T. D. (2014). Interviewing children. *Annual Review of Law and Social Science, 10,* 73–89.

Perry, B. D. (2009). Examining child maltreatment through a neurodevelopmental lens: Clinical applications of the neurosequential model of therapeutics. *Journal of Loss and Trauma, 14,* 240–255.

Spehar, C. (2015). Playful pathways to a resilient mindset: A play journey to triumph over adversity. In D. A. Crenshaw, R. Brooks, & S. Goldstein (Eds.), *Play therapy interventions to enhance resilience* (pp. 218–244). New York: Guilford Press.

Starr, C. R., & Ferguson, G. M. (2012). Sexy dolls, sexy grade schoolers?: Media and maternal influences on young girls' self sexualization. *Sex Roles, 67*(7), 463–476.

Sue, D. W. (2010). *Microaggressions in everyday life: Race, gender, and sexual orientation.* New York: Wiley.

Tishelman, A., & Geffner, R. (2010). Forensic, cultural, and systems issues in child sexual abuse cases—Part 2: Research and practitioner issues. *Journal of Child Sex Abuse, 19,* 609–617.

van der Kolk, B. (2006). Clinical implications of neuroscience research in PTSD. *Annals of the New York Academy of Sciences, 40,* 1–17.

van der Kolk, B. (2015). *The body keeps the score: Brain, mind, and body in the healing of trauma.* New York: Viking Press.

Art Therapy Approaches to Facilitate Verbal Expression

Getting Past the Impasse

Cathy A. Malchiodi

As described in Chapter 1, sensory-based, action-oriented approaches are effective ways to facilitate expression of personal narratives while allowing young clients to regain control and reestablish emotional regulation. Art expression is one specific sensory-based, action-oriented approach that gives children a way to tell stories, convey metaphoric content, and present worldviews, both through what is presented in their images and through their own responses to their creations (Malchiodi, 1998, 2007, 2015). The narrative qualities found in children's art and possibilities for facilitating storytelling offer therapists another way of understanding young clients in treatment. Through expanding the range of how children can express their "storied" lives in treatment, the process of reparation naturally integrates the richness of sensory-based experiences, nonverbal gestures, and visual symbols as pathways to narratives.

This chapter briefly introduces the foundations of art therapy with children with an emphasis on art-based intervention as a source of communication and personal narratives. While there are many types of art media that children can use to express themselves, the discussion focuses primarily on drawing because it is a medium with which many practitioners are familiar. Finally, several approaches to work with children who "clam up" or have reached an impasse in therapy are presented along with brief case vignettes to illustrate principles in practice.

ART THERAPY AND CHILDREN

Art therapy can be defined as the application of the visual arts and the creative process within a therapeutic relationship to support, maintain, and improve the psychosocial, physical, cognitive, and spiritual health of individuals of all ages (Malchiodi, 2007, 2013). It is an approach that is part of a larger array of creative arts therapies (art, music, dance/movement, and drama) that emerged as distinct forms of treatment in the mid-20th century. In addition, play therapists, counselors, and psychologists often use art-based approaches with clients, particularly with children, to help them communicate feelings and experiences through developmentally appropriate action-oriented strategies. In fact, art therapy and play therapy approaches often overlap since each is a creative, action-oriented form of therapy that demands participation and sensory self-expression.

Child art therapy has a long history in mental health, health care, rehabilitation, and education (Malchiodi, 2014b; Rubin, 2005; Shore, 2013). It is often applied in conjunction with various theoretical approaches including psychoanalytic, object relations, humanistic, cognitive-behavioral, and integrative, expressive arts applications (Malchiodi, 2012b). In particular, it is used to address trauma because it allows young clients to express themselves nonverbally. For example, in the aftermath of the terrorist attacks in September 11, 2001, and more recently in intervention with survivors of mass violence such as the Sandy Hook Elementary School shooting (Loumeau-May, Seibel, Pelicci-Hamilton, & Malchiodi, 2015), art therapy played a key role in helping children communicate complex reactions to mass trauma. For those who have been abused or violated, art expression is a widely accepted way to communicate feelings and experiences without words. It is also used to address a variety of emotional, cognitive, and physical challenges, including attention-deficit/hyperactivity disorder (Safran, 2012), autism (Gabriels & Gaffey, 2013), and medical illnesses (Beebe, 2013; Council, 2012) as a form of nonverbal, developmentally appropriate intervention.

In applying art therapy to work with children who are reticent to talk, there are two overarching goals: to assist children in externalizing thoughts, feelings, events, and worldviews through artistic expression and subsequent storytelling; and to help therapists develop an effective relationship with children that supports reparation through the creative process of making art. Art therapy is essentially a relational intervention that offers opportunities for connection through active participation between therapist and young client (Malchiodi, 2014a); in other words, it is essential that helping professionals who purposively integrate art activities into treatment understand that it is the relationship, not any specific technique or activity, that ultimately promotes change and well-being in children. In addition, there is no single art-based method that will "get pass the impasse" in therapy with a child who clams up. Rather, it is the appropriate and strategic introduction of creative expression along with the therapist's relational skills that form effective interventions and encourage children's narratives.

CAN CHILDREN'S STORIES
BE INTERPRETED FROM ART EXPRESSIONS?

Helping professionals often wonder whether they can interpret what children are thinking or feeling solely from their drawings or art expressions in an effort to bypass the need for verbal communication. Interpreting children's art expressions from one's own intuition or information found in projective drawing literature can be counterproductive, mainly because the existing literature on symbolic content in children's art is generally unreliable or invalid (Malchiodi, 1998, 2014b). On the other hand, children's creative expressions do convey their unique personalities, life experiences, memories, perceptions, emotions, and worldviews. Typical developmental characteristics, particularly from the ages of 6 (schematic expression) through 11 years (early realism), are identifiable and may be influenced by exposure to traumatic events (Malchiodi, 1998, 2014a). But there really are no universal symbols or graphic qualities that consistently can be said to have specific meanings or can be related to specific disorders; each child's story, as told through art, is unique and often idiosyncratic.

To explain the challenge of understanding children's drawings, this passage found in Antoine de Saint Exupéry's story *The Little Prince* (1943) provides a good example of how children are affected by adults' interpretation and even well-intended response to their creative expressions:

> Once when I was six years old I saw a magnificent picture in a book about the primeval forest. It was a picture of a boa constrictor in the act of swallowing an animal. . . . In the book it said: "Boa constrictors swallow their prey whole, without chewing it." After some work with a colored pencil I succeeded in making my first drawing. I showed my masterpiece to the

grown-ups, and asked them whether the drawing frightened them. But they answered: "Frighten? Why should anyone be frightened by a hat?" (pp. 3–4)

The story's narrator decided not to draw again because adults continually misunderstood his pictures; it is difficult for therapists to see children's art expressions with anything but adult eyes and standards. However, when working with children who come to treatment with histories of crises, loss, adverse events, or trauma, most therapists naturally seek to find meaning in their images, particularly when children are reticent to talk. This need to explain images is genuine; when viewing what seems like emotional pain or stories of crises or trauma, helping professionals naturally want to relate the contents of these images to what may be occurring in children's lives. Even the most expert practitioners can find themselves intuitively placing specific meaning and significance on characteristics of children's art expressions, especially when children are troubled or depressed and hesitant to speak about what is painful or confusing. In brief, it is important to maintain a "beginner's mind" when looking at young clients' art; an objective stance, even when one has a pretty good hunch about the content, respects the child's pace of communication both through images and language. It also encourages the use of open-ended questions (discussed later in this chapter) that provide children with a necessary sense of control in terms of conversation and self-expression.

SETTING THE STAGE FOR TALKING: SELF-REGULATION, CONNECTION, AND CONFIDENCE

Perry (2016) notes that the first step to any therapeutic success is lower-brain regulation, followed by moving sequentially through higher levels of the brain as improvements occur. He proposes "regulate, relate, reason" as the critical order in therapeutic intervention, education, and successful parenting and caregiving with children. In brief, until children can regulate (feel calm and safe), they are unlikely to be able to successfully relate to helping professionals. Once they are able to relate, children are then capable of engaging in higher-level cognitive processes necessary for not only problem solving, but also communicating perspectives and worldviews. In Perry's view, repetitive interventions emerge from positive, nurturing interactions with adults and trusted peers and capitalize on patterned, sensory-based activities such as dance, movement, yoga, drumming, and similar experiences. This sequential strategy is particularly important for young clients with persistent hyperactivation; it is necessary first to address the overwhelming fear and anxieties in these children before positive relationships can be established and to support and strengthen their cognitive capacities.

Similarly, in order to set the stage for meaningful and productive communication with children in art therapy, I generally focus art-based intervention in specific three areas: calm, connection, and confidence (Malchiodi, 2015). *Calm* refers to the basic goal of all treatment to help the individual learn to self-regulate and feel safe while developing skills to reduce stress when faced with upsetting events. I find that art therapy with children is very similar in some ways to mindfulness, a process of focusing on the present, because engagement in art expression often reduces anxiety and slows down the body's hyperactivation. Art materials can have a calming effect on young clients; depending on the child, constructing, painting, or working with clay in a repetitive way can help a child begin the process of self-regulation necessary to experience a sense of calm necessary to developing a trusting relationship with the therapist.

Providing art-based experiences that support self-regulation are an important foundation for "talk." As previously mentioned, regulation is necessary for both a relationship to occur and for reasoning (cognitive capacity) to be possible; in order for children to be able to tap the cognitive capacities needed to communicate stories through language. In addition, there is some evidence that the relaxing, diversionary qualities of art expression are helpful in supporting the flow of conversation (Gross & Haynes, 1998; Lev-Weisel & Liraz, 2007); studies demonstrate that children actively engaged in drawing are more likely to verbally relate details and memories than children who are asked to just talk. Providing a pleasurable hands-on activity like drawing may help a fearful child, for example, feel more at ease in talking with a helping professional.

Connection is the second key element in successful helping relationships; social support and positive attachment are central to resilience throughout childhood and the lifespan. While connection can be established in a variety of ways during the art therapy process, one specific way is the strategic use of the therapist's "third hand." Art therapist Edith Kramer (1993) is credited with the term "the third hand" and its application to clinical work. In brief, the third hand refers to the art therapist's use of suggestion, metaphors, or other techniques to enhance the individual's progress in therapy. What Kramer calls the third hand in art therapy echoes what Siegel (2010) refers to as "mindsight," a capacity for insight (knowing what one feels) and empathy (knowing what others feel). Thus, third-hand interventions are provided nonintrusively (with insight and empathy) so that the therapist does not change the content of the child's art expression or inadvertently influence the individual.

There are many ways the "third hand" is used in art therapy to encourage both verbal and nonverbal communication. For example, when working with a child client, I might begin a drawing for the child to complete as a way of establishing a relationship or communication. Other times, I might make art during the session alongside a client if it is therapeutically helpful, or I might even communicate something nonverbally through an art expression. These are moments of attunement, a relational dynamic that helps to build a healthy sense of self in children, and is a central feature in every caring relationship (Perry & Szalvitz, 2007).

Attunement is also the capacity to be able to read the nonverbal communication and rhythms of others. In other words, it is perceiving not only what individuals say, but also attending to eye signals, facial gestures, tone of voice, and even breathing rate, similar to what Porges (2011) proposes as part of the social engagement system. In art therapy, it also means attending to the content of images and nonverbal cues, as reflected in how well the therapist uses the third hand in response to the client's creative process. Because art therapy involves hands-on, sensory-based activities, it provides observational, responsive, and relational moments not necessarily found in talk therapy alone.

Connection is also established through authentic curiosity; this is possibly the most persuasive quality a therapist can have when it comes to children who are hesitant to speak. Introducing art expression as part of therapy sets the stage for curiosity because art images become an additional focus of interaction between therapist and child. As an art therapist, I always approach each session with excitement about what children will create, the surprises individuals bring to therapeutic encounters through their image making, and ultimately the detective story that all art expressions present. Just being interested in every part of a child's creative process and products communicates your genuine interest. In addition, as in any therapeutic relationship, the helping professional's noticeable belief in art-based methods they employ and their ability to project a charismatic personality (Brooks & Goldstein, 2015) are powerful motivating factors in both the establishment of connection as well as young clients' belief in treatment.

Finally, *confidence* is any experience that involves a sense of mastery that supports an internal locus of control and subsequently the belief that one can successfully address challenges. In art therapy, it is particularly important to help children feel in control of the creative process, supporting a pace that is within their "window of tolerance" (Siegel, 2012). In other words, art experiences that have some degree of challenge, but are not overwhelming, can help enhance self-efficacy and increase children's comfort levels with communication with the therapist.

It is also helpful to introduce art therapy and art expression as a process that children control in terms of pace and disclosure. In other words, during the first session I usually tell children that they "can tell as much or as little" as they want when participating in art therapy, and that it is perfectly okay not to say anything at all. I also offer that some children like to talk while drawing pictures or making things in the art therapy room and that I enjoy talking with children who come to art therapy sessions because I like learning more about them through their art. The latter is extremely important because if art therapy does not resonate as an approach with the therapist, children quickly sense a lack of enthusiasm for the process and that any art activities introduced may be just another "trick" to get information from them. Overall, my goal in building confidence and a sense of control is to help children clearly understand that the creative products made during art therapy sessions are not intended to be personality tests or evaluations, but that these expressions are part of a larger process to help them "feel better."

ENCOURAGING TALK THROUGH QUESTIONS

Children who experience positive attachment early in life and have good social support during times of stress or crisis generally have no problem talking about their creative expressions with helping professionals. In fact, when very young children first start to draw, they often come to expect that adults are interested in what they create and will ask them questions about their drawings or constructions. They will tell imaginative stories about their artworks without much prompting and are eager to share all sorts of details about with a parent, caregiver, or teacher.

For children who are challenged by emotional distress or have experienced insecure or disrupted attachment, the capacity to tell stories about art expressions may be difficult for emotional, developmental, or interpersonal reasons. The inventive narratives easily shared by their peers are not possible, and while they may be able to create with crayons, paint, or clay, these children may not know where to start when asked, "Can you tell me about your picture?" In this case, there are also some general questions that are possible ways to invite conversation about art expressions with many children (Malchiodi, 1997, 1998, 2014b; Steele & Malchiodi, 2012):

• *"What title would you give this picture or art? Tell me about what you made."* Or, *"What is going on in this drawing?"* These are obviously broad questions that can be helpful as openings to communication and dialogue.

• *"How do the people, animals, or objects in this drawing or artwork feel?"* With children who seem reticent to speak, I often start with queries that allow them to respond through elements in a drawing or art expression, rather than directly about themselves. This third-person approach permits children to use projection just as they would with a puppet or figures in a sandtray; for children who are understandably distressed due to interpersonal violence or trauma, this strategy can provide a sense of control over what they communicate. When I ask children about how inanimate objects such as a tree or a rock feel, children may think the therapist, in fact, has serious problems, but I often preface the question by offering, "Let's pretend that car, tree, house, or rock has feelings." If there are just colors, shapes or lines in a drawing, I might ask, "How does this shape (color or line) feel today?

• *"How do the figures in your artwork (drawing, clay constructions, painting, or collage) feel about one another? If they could speak, what would they say to each other?"* While these questions are related to emotions, they also may help a child express a story about a drawing or other art expression. To engage the child, the therapist may also pretend to be the voice of one of the figures, animals, or objects in art expression and ask the child to speak for another figure in the drawing. This approach is similar to that of play therapy when using toys or sandtray figures in a dialogue with each other.

• *"Can I ask the little girl, little boy, man, woman, cat, dog, house, tree, and so forth, something?"* This line of questioning encourages the child to imagine statements that various components of the art expression might make.

Most of these questions use a third-person approach rather than ask children to relate first-person stories. In particular, children who clam up often respond more positively to a less direct approach because it provides an added layer of safety and distance (confidence), but allows them to be the experts (control) in relating meaning about their art expressions. This is particularly true for children who are reticent to speak because they have lost trust in adults who may have hurt, betrayed, or abandoned them in the past or if they believe that they need to maintain secrecy about a family member or distressing event.

ENCOURAGING TALK THROUGH PROPS

For other children, introducing some sort of a prop such as a puppet, mask, or toy to act out an answer or tell a story. In this case, the therapist can simply ask, "Would you like to use a toy or puppet who can talk for you?" Or "Can one of these puppets answer the question I asked?" In addition to introducing play therapy props, an expressive arts approach may also be helpful. For example, dramatic enactment, movement, or sound, with or without props, can engage some children; the energy that it takes to communicate in this way can stimulate a conversation and at the very least add sensory-based experiences to the session. I often ask young clients, "Let's try something for fun. Can you show me through a movement what that person in your drawing would do if he could move? If he could make a sound, what kind of sound would he make?" Or "Can you show me through a movement what happens next?" For those children who are hesitant to get up and move, hand puppets are an alternative and can make movements or sounds.

Finally, sometimes the therapist needs a prop or two to encourage storytelling about artwork to get children to talk. For example, I keep what would now be considered an old-fashioned tape recorder on hand; it uses cassette tapes and has the advantage of a hand-held microphone that reinforces the experience of an interview. It has the benefit of recording stories verbatim and most children like the playback feature so they can hear their own voices and what was said. It also allows me to wonder out loud about the story details when we play back the recording. Even shy or quiet children get excited, curious, and increasingly animated when they see this contraption and experience a therapist who is willing to ham it up while dramatizing an interview with a child about a drawing or other creation. Similarly, some children may respond to seeing themselves on film; with the many possibilities from small video cameras to tablets and smartphones, it can be another option for conducting an "interview" about artwork and then watching and reacting to it during playback (with child assent and parent permission).

STARTING A CONVERSATION ABOUT THE "UNUSUAL"

In looking at any child's artwork, I generally ask myself, "What seems unusual, emphasized, or important in this image or object?" This observation can be used as a point of conversation and dialogue; it can be particularly effective with preschool and school-age children, who sometimes emphasize elements of their drawings through size or characteristics. Here is one example that describes how a child's drawing with an unusual feature became an effective starting point for dialogue between the girl and myself and led to the disclosure of an abusive situation in her home.

Case Example: Stacia

Stacia was an 8-year-old girl who was referred by child protective services (CPS) for art and play therapy for possible sexual abuse after her classroom teacher reported what she considered inappropriate sexual behavior at school. Her social worker suspected that Stacia had been abused by a family member, but she was selectively mute, especially when asked "who hurt you" or "who touched you." Her parents were cooperative with protective services, but English was their second language and the social worker who handled the case did not feel that they really understood why CPS was concerned about their daughter.

Like some children within her age range, Stacia depicted an X-ray view of her home with her in it. When I asked about the house drawing, Stacia eagerly explained that the house had two floors and pointed out that on the second floor there were several bedrooms and two bathrooms. On the first floor was a family room with a large television and a kitchen with what Stacia said was a refrigerator. It was very detailed and colorful; it struck me as unusual and large for its size in comparison to the rest of the drawing's contents. The television also seemed quite prominent, but of course many families have large flat-screen TVs in their homes. At the start of the session, I asked Stacia a couple of general questions of her picture and she politely responded to each of my queries, but did not volunteer any stories beyond what I specifically asked her. I then pointed out the refrigerator that was prominent in her drawing. Stacia's whole composure began to change in that instant, as if I had finally recognized what was important to her in the picture. She told me at that point that everyone in the family went to the refrigerator in the kitchen before they left the house in the morning.

Following Stacia's lead and mention of the routine activity in the kitchen, I asked her if she could name the people who went to the refrigerator before they left the house each day and what they took out of it. Stacia said her mother and father, who left the house first, took out milk and eggs for breakfast; her two older sisters, who went to high school, came to the kitchen next to make their lunches. When I asked who was left after that, there was an older brother who often overslept and was late for work; he rushed to the refrigerator to get a "red drink" (energy drink in a can) and left to catch a bus. Finally, when I asked, "So is anyone still at home besides you?" she quietly said that only she and her uncle, who was unemployed and stayed home to watch her.

While it became obvious that Stacia's uncle might indeed be the perpetrator, this first session led to additional art and play sessions that eventually confirmed he was sexually abusing her during the day after everyone else had left for work or school. As it turned out, the television in the drawing did play an important role in the eventual details of Stacia's experiences; the uncle turned it on for her to watch cartoons while he abused her. I learned from Stacia and her drawings and play activity that she "disappeared" (dissociated as an adaptive coping response) when her uncle was abusive. While her disclosure led to additional, long-term intervention, fortunately elements in Stacia's initial drawing helped her to tell "what happened" with important details to help me and her protective service worker to intervene.

REDIRECTING THE CONVERSATION

In the television series *Mad Men,* lead character Don Draper says, "If you don't like what's being said, change the conversation." This quote reminds me of another common impasse in child therapy—a young client who is stuck in a nonproductive narrative or artistic response and cannot, for whatever reason, move on to a more hopeful, reparative story that leads to recovery. While helping professionals unconditionally accept what children communicate during sessions, there are situations when children "get stuck" and cannot get past a particular story or memory while in treatment. In a positive sense, these children are not hesitant to talk and are actively engaged communicating with their therapists, but are really not getting any closer to resolving what is troubling them. They repetitively talk about what happened to them, what they witnessed, or what they encountered; they may even recreate a certain drawing or art expression during each therapy without feeling better afterwards. It may be a particular traumatic event or loss or other experience that becomes the focus of nonproductive perseveration or even obsession, creating a situation in which these young clients are unable to move to productive reframing and reparation. While time may resolve the repetition, most helping professionals understand that a child is not making progress and is, in fact, experiencing emotional pain and may even become retraumatized by retelling a story over a series of sessions.

Case Example: Josh

Josh, age 10, was referred to me by his dad, Craig, because of a car accident in which Josh's friend, Tom, also 10 years old, was admitted to the hospital because of his injuries. Josh and his father sustained minor bruises, but no serious injuries. The accident was the unfortunate result of a young woman who was distracted and ran a red light, hitting Craig's car.

At Craig's request, I made several home visits to work with Josh and his father about the trauma instead of at the office. Before my first home visit, Craig reported to me that Josh was obsessed with repeating the story of the accident and had even recreated the car crash in drawings he made at school; his teacher confirmed that Josh had become very distracted since the accident and was unable to concentrate on class activities. Josh also worried incessantly about Tom, even though he visited his friend in the hospital and at home and understood that he was recovering and would return to school soon.

When I initially met with Josh, I told him that it was okay to talk about what happened and that I would like to learn more about his experiences. Josh recounted the accident in great detail as well as what happened when he and his father followed the ambulance with Tom in it to the hospital and other important events associated with the car crash. He even asked me if I wanted him to repeat the story or had any questions. As Craig reported to me by phone, Josh's retelling of the accident never left him relieved, but in fact made him more anxious and sometimes even breathless. While the repetitive narration and drawings about the incident did not seem to be retraumatizing, they also were not helping Josh to feel relieved and self-regulated. In this case, it was important to consider ways to "change the conversation" without denying Josh the chance to tell his story and be heard.

In a subsequent meeting, Josh talked about the accident again and showed me "what happened" through several drawings about the major events during that day. I suggested to Josh that we ask his father to join us in the session if that was okay with him, explaining that I thought his father also might need to share in the storytelling because he might be upset about what happened on that day too. When Craig joined us, I explained that Josh and he shared an important story and that maybe it would help to make a special time to tell it and then, like placing a book on a bookshelf, to put it away until another time when it could be told again. Because Josh had created detailed drawings about the accident, those drawings would become part of the storytelling each time the story was told. At this juncture, Josh, Craig and I co-created a ritual for the telling of the "accident story" between this session and the next week. First, after the story was told, the drawings would be placed in a large envelope and put on a shelf (I pointed out one that had books and magazines on it in the living room). The envelope would stay there until it was time to talk about what happened again; Josh would also ask his father to retrieve the envelope from the bookshelf and have his father participate in the storytelling with him each time. I suggested that at this point it did not matter how many times the story was told, but that the ritual of the storytelling (father and son together, retrieving the envelope, sitting down to look at the drawings and tell the story, placing the drawings back in the envelope and putting it back on the shelf) was important.

During next few days, Craig and Josh followed the plan each night after dinner. When I arrived the next week for Josh's session, I again listened to the story and reviewed the drawings with Josh. But after the recounting of the accident, I asked him to tell me more about his friend Tom, who was about to return to school, something that pleased Josh. In particular, I asked him if he could show any photographs of himself and Tom together; as it turned out, there were quite a few to share because, as Josh said, "Tom and me hung out together a lot." I suggested that if it was okay with him and his father, we could add these photographs to the envelope for now and that perhaps he could make some new drawings at this session about some of things that he and Tom did together before the accident. In other words, I was actually asking him to create images of when the accident "was not happening" and also to include photographs of the memories about the many positive times Josh and Tom experienced together. While a few more sessions were necessary to redirect Josh away from the dominant trauma narrative, he also gradually became less focused on the story of the car accident. In part, his father's perseverance with reinforcing the limits of retelling the story and the storytelling ritual was extremely helpful. However, the integration of other experiences and events through images in the form of drawings and photos, along with storytelling, broadened the narrative to include the many positive things that Josh had in his life, especially with his friend Tom; the "conversation" moved away from the accident to positive talk that included good memories and thoughts about the future.

Introducing another art medium is another possible way to change or redirect a nonproductive narrative. Drawings are excellent means of telling stories, particularly sequential events or timelines. However, drawings are static expressions; that is, it is difficult to alter a drawing done in felt pen or crayons. Introducing a three-dimensional and malleable material or medium like modeling clay or Play-Doh opens up possibilities for making adaptations to a story through movement and rearranging elements; new objects or entities like helpers or first responders, for example, can be introduced to create new endings to stories or play out themes of rescue, recovery, and self-efficacy. Sandtrays provide another way to make images through arrangement of miniature figures that the child can easily move around and manipulate. In brief, the therapist can suggest elements to a child's story or ask, "If you moved that figure over here, what would be different about the story you have told me?" The point is to allow children to retell their stories, but also to strategically invite them to redirect the story through by the position or arrangement of objects in the sandtray or other media.

SEPARATING THE CHILD FROM THE PROBLEM

Narratives are a core element of most forms of psychotherapy and, as Michael White (White & Epston, 1990) proposes, they help individuals externalize problems from the person. In narrative therapy, this is summed up as "The problem is the problem, the person is not the problem." While narrative therapists speak of this phenomenon in terms of verbal storytelling or writing, art expression serves much the same function for children by externalizing their experiences, thoughts, and feelings through visual images. It can be a potent way of initiating the process of communication in therapy because it not only validates children's experiences, but it also helps them to put some distance between their problems and themselves. In other words, art expression helps in establishing that the problem, whether it's a troubling feeling, traumatic event or loss, or situation, is separate from the self.

About children's art expressions as forms of narrative therapy, Riley (2001) writes:

> The therapist can step into the child's drawings and let him/her teach the meaning of this visual narrative. The art is a form of personal externalization, an extension of oneself, a visual projection of thoughts or feelings. When art is accepted, honored, and validated by the therapist, the creator is (through identification with the art product) equally accepted, honored, and validated. The client, in this case a child, can better understand through these actions than through words that he/she has been confirmed and valued. When the problem or anxiety has been externalized by the child in a drawing, it is the perfect time to confront the problem-laden behavior and still validate the worth of the creator (the child artist). (p. 31)

In work with children who are reticent to talk, the goal of separating the problem from the person through art is twofold. First, it is key to establish an atmosphere where guilt, blame, and shame are alleviated. As an art therapist, one of my initial goals is to help children understand that the focus of our meetings is on supporting them in finding their strengths rather than seeking to identify what is "wrong with you" through their artwork. This is not only a narrative approach, it also reflects a trauma-informed expressive arts therapy perspective (Malchiodi, 2012c; Steele & Malchiodi, 2012) that emphasizes the inherent capacity of the individual to participate in treatment, influence the therapeutic process, and literally "have a voice" in what happens.

The second goal involves inviting children to be active in solving the problem at hand. Art therapy, expressive arts therapy, and play therapy have an advantage over talk therapy in separating the problem from person because they are action-oriented approaches that capitalize on children's expertise in arts and play. To encourage children to find a means of arts-based communication, the therapist can begin with invitations like:

"Sometimes things are hard to talk about, but there are other ways to share thoughts and feelings through a drawing or toy. What ways do you like?"

"What does the problem/event/worry look like to you? Can you show me in a drawing using colors, lines, and shapes? If you want, you can just pick a color that reminds you of the problem and make some marks on paper to show me what it looks like to you."

"Can you move your body in a way that shows me how it feels when the worry takes over?" Encouraging movement can be particularly good for children who may be hypoactive or withdrawn, or respond to stress with freeze reactions (as opposed to flight or fight).

"Using figures and objects in the sandtray, can you make a picture or a map of when the worry or problem takes over?"

In all cases, once children translate the worry or problem into something visual, they generally have an easier time talking about it. One particularly effective way to encourage externalization of problems or worries that children and teenagers decline to discuss is through introducing an evocative art-based activity. Masks are one such activity because they often result in self-portraits and have the added benefit of allowing their creators to use them to "speak" in a way similar to a puppet. A plain paper mask that can be painted and embellished with a variety of colorful, tactile materials (glitter glue, feathers, beads, ribbons) invites participation even with the most reticent children; it is also a particularly good way to generate narratives with adolescents who enjoy working with masks to express what may otherwise be left unspoken, as described in this brief case example.

Case Example: Arianna

When I first met 14-year-old Arianna, she was referred to an expressive arts therapy resiliency program I facilitated for children and families in the U.S. military. She was enrolled in an expressive arts group specifically for teens because her family felt that she might benefit from creative activities since she was hesitant to talk in counseling sessions and becoming more withdrawn in school. Her parents understandably worried that Arianna might be depressed, and her father was concerned that his unpredictable multiple deployments and responsibilities away from home were contributing to her recent withdrawal; he felt that his daughter was previously an outgoing and highly communicative preteenager and now suddenly seemed preoccupied and disengaged from her parents and siblings.

In fact, when Arianna first joined the expressive arts group, I could barely get her to introduce herself to the other participants. Although she seemed to enjoy the activities, she always shook her head to let me know that her answer was "no" when asked if she wanted to share something about her artwork each week. While I tried various strategies and questions to invite Arianna to talk in the group or privately with me, I was not making much progress. The turning point in Arianna's participation came about during a session focused on using a lifelike paper face mask to communicate two "self-portraits." The teenagers were asked to paint and embellish the outside of their masks in order to show "how you believe others see you"; on the inside of the masks, they were asked to depict "what others do not know about you and how you really feel inside."

Arianna quickly became engaged in decorating her mask, carefully painting the outside to look like herself—an image of an attractive, yet serious-looking adolescent female and an accurate reflection of herself as others saw her. The inside of her mask was quite different; Arianna assembled magazine clippings of text including "no return" and "lonely" in addition to images of storm clouds, tears, and anger. It seemed to externalize the unspoken thoughts and feelings Arianna had yet to speak about in the resiliency group. But fortunately when the group participants were invited to display their masks on a table so everyone could view them, Arianna immediately looked at me and asked, "Aren't we going to talk about our masks?" Each week the group spent part of the session talking about their art, but until this moment she declined to speak about her artwork or respond to any of the other creations. It was obvious that this particular process had tapped into something that she finally wanted to share.

As the group discussion about each mask proceeded, Arianna chose to hold up her mask next to one side of her face and talked about the outside as "what I think I look like to others" and how she was "pretty shy," and liked to listen to music and write in her journal at home in her bedroom. When I asked her if she would like to say anything about the inside of the mask, she quickly flipped it over to reveal her collage images and text and said, "I don't know about everyone else here, but I don't understand why he [her father] want to put himself in danger over and over." In a softer voice, she added, "I really want to tell him to stay home the next time." Any helping professional who has worked with military and their families knows that what Arianna said is one of the most difficult experiences to speak out loud, often for reasons of guilt or shame; military children often believe they must stay strong for their parents and particularly the parent who is deployed to a combat zone or other dangerous situation. This moment of disclosure confirmed at least some of the struggles that Arianna had kept silent; it also served as a catalyst for a larger discussion within the group about what is a difficult issue for many young people in military families. Most important, it was a relief to Arianna's parents, who were understandably afraid that their daughter was perhaps depressed or even suicidal because of her very real "mask" of silence. While this was just the first stage of addressing Arianna's fears about her father's multiple deployments, fortunately this particular art-based activity allowed her to speak and reinforced that she could share her concerns with me, with peers in the resiliency group, and with her parents.

CONCLUSION

There is no one way to go about getting children to talk about their art expressions during therapy, just as there is no one surefire method to encourage storytelling through play or other action-oriented techniques. How each child presents during treatment is a complex mix of personality, temperament, past experiences, current situation, the art-based approach, and the relationship between therapist and child client. Introducing the opportunity for creative expression is, however, a strategy that opens up many possibilities with children who clam up during treatment because visual images are natural sources for storytelling. It also provides a rich terrain to explore with children through our questions and responses to art products; the multidimensional qualities of artistic creations, such as Arianna's mask, can evoke personal narratives that may otherwise remain unspoken. Finally, while art may speak for children without words, it also has the potential to make words possible even for those young clients who have reached an impasse in treatment by making it once again possible not only to be witnessed, but also be heard.

FIVE RECOMMENDED PRACTICES

1. Be curious about every element in children's creative work. Your enthusiasm about the creative process and your genuine interest is key to encouraging storytelling.

2. Establish and support calm (self-regulation and safety), connection (secure relationship and trust), and confidence (sense of mastery and self-efficacy). This will establish an atmosphere not only for creative expression, but also for trust in verbal disclosure.

3. Introduce art expression as a way to help children learn that the person is not the problem—the problem is the problem. By reinforcing that creative expression helps to separate the problem from the child, the child becomes actively engaged in not only finding solutions, but also in talking with the therapist about how to do so.

4. Use questions that encourage third-person responses. Allowing children to speak through their drawings or other art expressions, rather than directly about themselves, is a good option for those who may be reticent to speak about particularly difficult emotions, circumstances, events, or memories.

5. Use a variety of art-based approaches and media not only to encourage creative expression, but also to stimulate narratives. Not every child or adolescent responds to drawing as a way to tell stories; be knowledgeable and flexible about additional art-based approaches to evoke personal narratives based on the client's preferences and personality.

REFERENCES

Beebe, A. (2013). Art therapy with children who have asthma. In C. Malchiodi (Ed.), *Art therapy and health care* (pp. 79–91). New York: Guilford Press.

Brooks, R., & Goldstein, R. (2015). The power of mindsets: Guideposts for a resilience-based treatment approach. In D. Crenshaw, R. Brooks, & S. Goldstein (Eds.), *Play therapy interventions to enhance resilience* (pp. 3–31). New York: Guilford Press.

Council, T. (2012). Medical art therapy with children. In C. Malchiodi (Ed.), *Handbook of art therapy* (2nd ed., pp. 222–240). New York: Guilford Press.

de Saint-Exupéry, A. (1943). *The little prince*. New York: Harcourt Brace Jovanavich.

Gabriels, R., & Gaffey, L. (2013). Art therapy with children on the autism spectrum. In C. Malchiodi (Ed.), *Handbook of art therapy* (2nd ed., pp. 205–221). New York: Guilford Press.

Gross, J., & Haynes, H. (1998). Drawing facilitates children's verbal reports of emotionally laden events. *Journal of Experimental Psychology, 4*, 163–179.

Kramer, E. (1993). *Art as therapy with children*. Chicago: Magnolia Street.

Lev-Weisel, R., & Liraz, R. (2007). Drawings versus narratives: Drawing as a tool to encourage verbalization in children whose fathers are drug abusers. *Clinical Child Psychology and Psychiatry, 12*(1), 65–75.

Loumeau-May, L., Siebel, E., Pellicci-Hamilton, M., & Malchiodi, C. A. (2015). Art therapy as an intervention for mass violence. In C. A. Malchiodi (Ed.), *Creative interventions with traumatized children* (2nd ed., pp. 94–125). New York: Guilford Press.

Malchiodi, C. A. (1997). *Breaking the silence: Art therapy with children from violent homes* (2nd ed.). New York: Taylor & Francis.

Malchiodi, C. A. (1998). *Understanding children's drawings*. New York: Guilford Press.

Malchiodi, C. A. (2007). *The art therapy sourcebook*. New York: MacMillan.

Malchiodi, C. A. (2012a). Art therapy and the brain. In C. Malchiodi (Ed.), *Handbook of art therapy* (2nd ed., pp. 17–25). New York: Guilford Press.

Malchiodi, C. A. (2012b). *Handbook of art therapy* (2nd ed.). New York: Guilford Press.

Malchiodi, C. A. (2012c). Trauma-informed art therapy and sexual abuse. In P. Goodyear-Brown (Ed.), *Handbook of child sexual abuse* (pp. 341–354). Hoboken, NJ: Wiley.

Malchiodi, C. A. (2013). Introduction to art therapy in health care settings. In C. Malchiodi (Ed.), *Art therapy and health care* (pp. 1–12). New York: Guilford Press.

Malchiodi, C. A. (2014a). Art therapy, attachment and parent–child dyads. In C. A. Malchiodi & D. Crenshaw (Eds.), *Creative arts and play therapy for attachment problems* (pp. 52–66). New York: Guilford Press.

Malchiodi, C. A. (2014b). Creative arts therapy approaches to attachment issues. In C. A. Malchiodi & D. A. Crenshaw (Eds.), *Creative arts and play therapy for attachment problems* (pp. 3–18). New York: Guilford Press.

Malchiodi, C. A. (2015). Calm, connection and confidence: Using art therapy to enhance resilience in traumatized children. In D. A. Crenshaw, R. Brooks, & S. Goldstein (Eds.), *Play therapy interventions to enhance resilience* (pp. 126–145). New York: Guilford Press.

Perry, B. D. (2016). *Self-regulation: The second core strength*. Retrieved on July 3, 2016, from *http://teacher.scholastic.com/professional/bruceperry/self_regulation.htm*.

Perry, B. D., & Szalvitz, M. (2007). *The boy who was raised as a dog*. New York: Basic Books.

Porges, S. (2011). *The polyvagal theory: Neurophysiological foundations of* emotions, attachment, communication and regulation. New York: Norton.

Riley, S. (2001). *Group process made visible*. New York: Taylor & Francis.

Rubin, J. (2005). *Child art therapy* (2nd ed.). Hoboken, NJ: Wiley.

Safran, D. (2012). An art therapy approach to attention-deficit/hyperactivity disorder. In C. Malchiodi (Ed.), *Handbook of art therapy* (2nd ed., pp. 192–204). New York: Guilford Press.

Shore, A. (2013). *A practitioner's guide to child art therapy*. New York: Routledge.

Siegel, D. (2010). *Mindsight: The new science of personal transformation*. New York: Norton.

Siegel, D. (2012). *The developing mind: How relationships and the brain interact to shape who we are* (2nd ed.). New York: Guilford Press.

Steele, W., & Malchiodi, C. A. (2012). *Trauma-informed practices with children and adolescents*. New York: Routledge.

White, M., & Epston, D. (1990). *Narrative means to therapeutic ends*. New York: Norton.

Animal Assisted Play Therapy
with Reticent Children

With a Little Help from Friends

Risë VanFleet
Tracie Faa-Thompson

For many years, we worked with reticent children using nondirective play therapy and Filial Therapy (FT) to address the basic emotional and social needs of children who didn't talk, or who didn't talk much. These approaches were generally successful, and we still use them as a means of helping children to meet their needs for a sense of control, work through their fears and emotional challenges, and establish stronger attachment relationships. Even so, these methods generally took a number of sessions followed by gradual improvement in their engagement in therapy. For children who felt unsafe with human adults, it could take even longer. When children were reluctant to engage in play therapy, even with nonverbal and symbolic play, it could take time for them to experience the acceptance of the play sessions and to feel safe enough to open up.

Then along came some individuals who were willing participants in our play therapy work who were able to bring about rather dramatic results with children who remained quiet or unengaged for various reasons. These "individuals" were dogs and horses, primarily, as well as cats, rabbits, and even fish! While both of the authors of this chapter have incorporated animals in our therapeutic work for many years, the idea of integrating specially selected and prepared animals into play therapy evolved gradually, and independently, for both of us. By the time we met and compared notes about 10 years ago, we knew that Animal Assisted Play Therapy™ (AAPT) had tremendous potential to help many clients, of all ages and with many different problems, in ways not yet fully understood or explored.

Nowhere was the potential assistance of animals in play therapy more obvious than with children who clammed up—children who felt unsafe entrusting therapists or anyone else with their inner struggles and pain. Their reasons for being cautious were many. Some had developmental and/or communication difficulties; others had been abused and had lost all trust; still others were shy and self-conscious; and some simply found that remaining silent was one way to control an uncontrollable world swirling about them.

Kirrie's (RV's primary play therapy dog for a decade) first client was a 13-year-old boy who had a long and horrible history with abusive caregivers. He had significant trauma and had never experienced a healthy attachment relationship until his current foster placement. He had had bad experiences in therapy, where therapists prodded him to "open up" or "speak up," with emphasis on his verbal behavior and little attention to the feelings that were driving him to remain silent. Efforts to engage even in small talk with him resulted in his hiding his face behind pillows. He looked down and said little. He had made strides with a play/filial therapist prior to receiving AAPT, but his therapist felt they had reached a plateau beyond which it was difficult for him to move. When his therapist went on medical leave, I first held several play sessions with him that went well, but I could see his difficulty in making conversation about even neutral topics. He expressed himself well in a symbolic fashion during a multimodal approach using nondirective play therapy, cognitive-behavioral play therapy, and FT with his current foster parent, but it was clear that he had more that he wanted and needed to express. His lack of trust of all humans held him back. When we began the AAPT sessions, he had an almost immediate transformation. Our focus was on doing things with Kirrie, and he began speaking animatedly to the dog and to me. The final blocks to communication seemed to lift, and he was able to relax enough to express and work through even more in the AAPT sessions, and he was able to engage in conversation with me, and subsequently, even more with his foster mother. The shift was noticeable to his caseworkers and teachers as well.

This type of shift for reticent children is not unusual when animals are included appropriately in therapy. In the sections that follow, AAPT is described, including the mechanisms that seem to work to help children who clam up feel safer and more engaged in the process. Case examples featuring dogs and horses illustrate AAPT with this population of children and teens.

DESCRIPTION OF AAPT

AAPT fully integrates the practice of play therapy with animal-assisted therapy (AAT). Animals are incorporated into the sessions in playful ways designed to help clients accomplish their therapeutic goals. The playfulness can take different forms, from the therapist's demeanor and ability to facilitate and debrief sessions in a lighthearted manner to fully engaged play activities that clients and animals participate in. Attention is paid to the clients' therapeutic goals as well as the well-being of the animals involved. It is a basic principle of AAPT that the animals must enjoy the work rather than merely tolerate it. There are forms of AAPT that are used with clients across the lifespan for a wide range of developmental, clinical, and interpersonal problems. It can be used with individual clients, families, and groups. AAPT is more fully described in other resources (VanFleet, 2008; VanFleet & Faa-Thompson, 2010, 2014, 2015a, 2015b, 2015c, 2017; VanFleet, Fine, O'Callaghan, Mackintosh, & Gimeno, 2015). This chapter focuses on its application with children and adolescents who have difficulty opening up in the therapy process.

COMPETENCIES REQUIRED FOR THE ETHICAL USE OF AAPT

AAPT is a complex intervention requiring substantial preparation. The animals involved must be carefully selected, not only for their stable personalities, but especially for their sociable and playful characteristics. While traditionally quiet and docile therapy dogs can be employed, AAPT permits more active animals to take part as well. It is important that when clients enter the venue in which AAPT occurs that the animals approach them with interest and curiosity. In the case of dogs, especially, and to a lesser extent with horses and cats, training is needed to ensure that the animal is under the behavioral control of the therapist. This does not mean that the therapist is *controlling*, but that the animal is able to behave as needed during the session. In fact, well-behaved but spirited animals who are honored for their uniqueness are ideal. The only way to accomplish this is by developing a mutually respectful and fun relationship between therapists and the animals. This type of relationship provides an important metaphor for therapy, serving as a model of the type of relationship the client can expect with the therapist as well as an example of the humane and compassionate treatment of animals. Creating a healthy alliance between therapist and animal takes time, patience, humility, and considerable knowledge of ethology, positive training methods, and fluency in reading and understanding animal body language.

It is increasingly common to hear about therapists who have a nice dog, cat, horse, rabbit, or other animal who decide to involve the animal in their work. This raises serious scope of practice ethical concerns. AAPT is simply not as easy as some seem to think. There are huge responsibilities that fall on the shoulders of the therapists, and they must be able to conduct quality therapy while attending to the subtle signals and needs of the animals. Risk management is accomplished by developing competencies in many aspects of animal handling and welfare, and knowing how to creatively blend the needs of the animals with the goals of therapy. There are countless possibilities after one develops these competencies, but they, too, take time. Just as one would not decide to practice hypnosis based on an online course, one should not decide to practice AAPT without substantial training with a strong hands-on component and supervision of actual sessions. One of the most common reactions of highly experienced play therapists when first conducting AAPT is how challenging it is to attend to the many variables and relationships operating simultaneously within the session.

A full description of AAPT can be found in a number of books, chapters, and articles (VanFleet, 2008; VanFleet & Faa-Thompson, 2010, 2014, 2015a, 2015b, 2015c, 2017; VanFleet et al., 2015). The International Institute for Animal Assisted Play Therapy™ (*www.iiaapt. org*) offers training, supervision, and certification in AAPT at several levels of expertise.

Mechanisms

There are a number of ways that AAPT can be valuable for children who clam up. The primary ones are listed below; more detailed descriptions of mechanisms of treatment can be found in other resources (Chandler, 2012; Fine, 2015; Parish-Plass, 2013; VanFleet, 2008, 2015a; VanFleet & Faa-Thompson, 2017).

Children's Interest in Animals

Melson (2001), Melson and Fine (2015), and Jalongo (2014) have studied and summarized the research pertaining to children's interest in animals. It is well documented that children throughout the world are very interested in animals—they like to see them, interact with them, draw pictures of them, hear stories about them, and even dream of them. It seems a developmental mainstay to attend to animals. Some have suggested that animals provide an important connection with the natural world, and interventions based in natural environments are gaining ground as children increasingly lead indoor lives (Louv, 2008; VanFleet, 2015b). A wise therapist seeks to understand the things that are important to children, and because animals seem prevalent, the incorporation of animals through AAPT or symbolically through therapeutic stories (Sheppard, 1998), sandtray figures, puppets, art interventions (Malchiodi, 2015), and other methods makes developmental sense. For reticent children, the presence of animals or animal symbols provides familiarity and the potential message that the setting has been designed with their interests in mind.

Authenticity, Reactions, and Projection

In AAPT, practitioners avoid "overtraining" the animal partners. The animals are not only permitted, but encouraged, to be who they are. This means that the animals do not always act in ways that the client or the therapist might desire, even if they have been carefully selected and prepared for this role. Sometimes they walk away; dogs might occasionally seem to forget their training cues and ignore human requests made of them; horses might choose to graze during the session. These are all natural behaviors, and therapists need not try to rid the animal of them in order to "stage" an intervention with a child. It is more important that the interaction be authentic.

The animals bring themselves and their own personalities and behaviors to the session. The therapist needs to have the flexibility and the insight and the clinical intervention skills to process the interaction with the client, based on the client's reactions, goals, and the form of AAPT being used. (AAPT can be delivered as a nondirective play therapy format or with varying degrees of structure in more directive formats [VanFleet, 2008; VanFleet et al., 2015; VanFleet, Sywulak, & Sniscak, 2010].) For example, if a child wants to interact with a horse, and the horse chooses to graze for a while, the therapist would not generally try to stop the horse from grazing. Clients might have very different reactions to that very natural behavior of the horse. One child might find it fascinating to hear the horse tear up the grass and munch on it. Another child simply will turn to something else. Yet another might be upset that the horse is ignoring him or her. In all of these cases, the children's reactions are authentic as well. This is where the practitioner still has to conduct therapy! The child who is upset with the horse's grazing might be prone to feelings of abandonment or rejection. The fact that this interaction arises and the child reacts in this manner provides the therapist with the opportunity to empathically respond to the child's feelings and help the child work through them—precisely what therapy is about! For children who are reluctant to be part of therapy, the interactions with the animals provide a conduit for expression and working through their difficulties. As Chandler (personal communication, April 25, 2015) has discussed, AAT in mental health treatment is made up of "relational moments," and the therapist's ability to recognize and process those moments with the clients is paramount. This is true of AAPT as well.

Social Lubrication Effects

Social lubrication is the term used for a phenomenon whereby one's interactions with an animal make it more possible to interact with other humans (Fine, 2015; VanFleet, 2008). Shy children who take their family companion dog for a walk seem to become less self-conscious and more willing to talk with others about the dog. The focus is on the animal, not the child, and the shyness drops away. In therapy with children who clam up, the social lubrication effect is one of the most important mechanisms that can be harnessed.

In therapy, having an animal partner in the process also provides social lubrication. While the child might be engaged primarily by the animal, it typically does not take long before the child begins to warm up to the therapist. The therapist, after all, has shared his or her animal with the child, and it is (or should be) obvious to the child that the therapist cherishes the animal and is pleased to share this experience with the child. In many cases by both authors, children who have said virtually nothing with other therapists or during initial sessions begin to talk spontaneously with the therapist within just a few sessions. The object of AAPT, just as with play therapy, is not to get the child to speak, but when a previously quiet child begins to talk, it signals a level of comfort that was not there before. It is also common for the nonverbal behaviors and postures of the child in AAPT to show interest, engagement, relaxation, and a willingness to take part more fully in the therapy experience, even when it is mostly through nonverbal expression.

Attachment and Relationship

Almost everything about AAPT, regardless of the specific modality employed, pertains to relationships. Clients learn to interact with the animals in a safe, friendly, and humane manner. They experience the animal's interest in them, and they learn to care for the animals. The therapist helps foster healthy attachment relationships between client and animal, and this can help clients learn the reciprocity so important in human relationships as well. Sessions can include attention to the animal's feelings and reactions, as well as empathy from the therapist for the client's responses. For children who are uneasy with other people or with the therapy process, the aforementioned social lubricant effects form a bridge to relationship building, first with the animals, and then with the therapist and other humans. Furthermore, group programs involving horses or dogs can encourage teamwork and consideration of others.

Confidence Building

Another way in which AAPT can help reticent children is by building their confidence. Children can learn to teach something new to a dog or how to handle themselves around horses who weigh half a ton or more. The *experience* with the animal is what matters, and seeing that one's own behaviors result in a response from the animal can be highly reinforcing and contribute to self-efficacy. Many shy or quiet children stand visibly taller, walk with greater confidence, and speak proudly of their accomplishments when working with the animals in AAPT: "Dad, I'm the one who came up with this idea!" is a common refrain as children or teens demonstrate some of the new behaviors they have taught the dog, or the skills they have in walking a horse through an obstacle course. Engaging in activities where they teach the animals new behaviors helps develop a sense of control, not of the animal, but of themselves.

Oxytocin Effects

The final mechanism to be covered in this chapter is that of the impact of oxytocin production when humans and animals interact. Olmert (2009, 2010) introduced the idea that oxytocin production might be at the root of the human–animal bond, and researchers have increasingly shown that is likely to be true (Morell, 2014; Olmert, 2010; Zak, 2014). Oxytocin, long known as the bonding neurohormone in mother–infant attachment, has been shown to increase when humans and dogs look at each other, interact, and play together. The increases generally are present for both humans and dogs. Research is continuing, but it seems likely that oxytocin production can be enhanced with certain types of interactions, and that finding eventually might help explain some of the therapeutic impact of animals in play therapy. Oxytocin production increases a range of positive emotional reactions, including trust, generosity, cooperation, and generally feeling better. It is believed to play an important role in the development of social relationships. For children who clam up in therapy, this oxytocin effect might provide the biological basis for some of the improvements noted consistently in the practice of AAPT. This has yet to be shown, but a number of research studies are underway that are likely to illuminate the role of oxytocin in animal-based interventions with mental health problems.

AAPT INTERVENTIONS

AAPT interventions can take many forms. In fact, AAPT can be merged with most major theories of psychological intervention, just as there are forms of play therapy that are grounded in these theories. There is a nondirective, or child-centered, form of AAPT in which the therapist sets up the playroom or establishes a play space with a variety of toys, and then allows the child to make most of the choices about what to play with and how to play. In AAPT, the child always has a choice about including the animal, but in nondirective AAPT, the child has more choice in how to include the animal. The therapist tries to respond in a nondirective, empathic, and accepting manner as much as possible, but can "give voice" to the animal through the various child-centered play skills. Nondirective AAPT is discussed in greater detail in VanFleet (2008, 2015a; VanFleet & Faa-Thompson, 2017).

Therapists can also use a range of directive AAPT methods, ranging from those with relatively low to fairly high structure. With directive approaches, the therapist typically suggests some activity that he or she believes will assist with client goal attainment. The levels of structure are described in more detail elsewhere (VanFleet et al., 2015). In short, with lightly structured activities, the therapist sets up the situation, then steps back and allows the client/s to participate in it without much input other than empathic listening and a debriefing at the end. Highly structured activities might involve showing the client how to teach the dog to learn a new trick or behavior, where the therapist plays a much more active role.

With quiet children, there is never an emphasis on the child's verbal language. In fact, the therapist would normally work with teachers, parents, and others in the child's life to ask them to avoid "trying to get the child to talk." The aim of this is to reduce the level of expectations and the amount of pressure on the child, and to return a sense of control to the child. With dogs, the therapist might teach the child two sets of cues for different behaviors. One is a gestural cue, where the child can use hand, arm or other body signals to communicate to the dog what is needed. Dogs generally learn gestural cues more readily than verbal ones anyway! The therapist also tells the child what the verbal cues for the same behaviors are, such as "Sit," "Down," "Roll over," or "Follow me." The child is then given a choice to use gestural or verbal cues. With all pressure taken off, many children eventually provide verbal cues as they become more involved with the dog and see how responsive the dog is to them. They often start with whispered cues accompanying the gestural cues, but the whispers often gain volume as the child's confidence and comfort increase. In another example, the therapist can set up an activity where the child tells something to the horse using whispers. The therapist stands back, providing space and respect for the child's need to have some privacy when talking with the horse. Gradually the therapist can become more involved, often using empathic listening in a quiet way until the child's comfort level increases.

Interventions in AAPT are limited only by therapists' imaginations, their knowledge of their animal partners, and their attunement with their clients. Some ideas are presented in VanFleet (2008), VanFleet and Faa-Thompson (2010, 2014, 2015a, 2015b, 2015c, 2017), and Van-Fleet et al. (2015). VanFleet and Faa-Thompson presently are writing a manual for practitioners with training in AAPT, *Animal Assisted Play Therapy Techniques*. Trotter (2012) has a book filled with activities that can be used therapeutically with horses and easily adapted to AAPT. The case examples in the next section include descriptions of a number of specific AAPT techniques.

CASE EXAMPLES

The following case illustrations show AAPT in action with children who clam up. Different types of reticence in children are included to demonstrate the application and flexibility of the AAPT modality.

Case 1: James

James was a 9-year-old boy who moved from a small rural school to a much larger middle school. Teachers reported that he was nonverbal at school and did not interact with anyone. He refused to eat, hid in the bushes, and attempted to gouge out his eyes if anyone tried to speak to or interact with him. He came to my (TF-T) equine program, Turn About Pegasus (TAP), to participate in a group of eight children between the ages of 9 and 12 who were viewed as vulnerable, socially isolated, and depressed. James was in the process of being evaluated for an autism spectrum disorder (ASD), which had not been recognized at his previous school.

Initially at the TAP program, James was nonverbal and gave little eye contact. It was difficult to know what he was getting out of the session; however, his parents said that he loved to come to it. The school people who accompanied him and the other children to the program said that he seemed like a different child when at TAP—jumping, smiling, and running about among the horses. He did appear to be happy there.

In the third session, an activity called Blindfolds was used. The children were asked to set up an obstacle course, and then they divided into teams of three children and one horse each. The purpose of the activity is to bring out issues of trust, relationships, and how difficult it can sometimes be to recognize whether someone is trustworthy. One child is blindfolded and must lead the horse through the obstacles. The other two children position themselves on either side of the blindfolded child, and they must tell the blindfolded child where to lead the horse to get through the obstacles. Without the blindfolded child knowing, one of them is designated as the "good influence" and the other takes on the role of the "bad influence." It was unknown how James would handle this activity because he had remained nonverbal to this point. Even so, the plan was to include him as much as possible.

The blindfolds used are similar to sleep masks, but they have funny-looking eyes on them. Some are animal eyes and others have big googly eyes. When the first child put on one of these blindfolds, the first thing everyone heard was a huge laugh from James. He pointed at the mask and laughed and laughed so much he had to turn away. Soon there were 18 people (children, TAP staff, and school support people) all laughing with him. Every time he turned back around to the group, he began laughing heartily all over again.

At that point, the loose horses came over to him. James then pointed to the person wearing the blindfold and asked the horses to look at his "friend." He leaned on Sailor, a big Gypsy Vanner, for support as he continued laughing. The activity took a long time as James struggled to look at his team members without laughing. From that point on, James became very verbal, talked about films he had watched in great detail, and asked many questions about the horses. It became clear that the horses meant a great deal to him, something that was difficult to ascertain previously.

James's verbal interactions transferred to school, and he began to talk with certain people. No longer did he hide in the bushes, and he stopped trying to gouge out his eyes. He made friends with two boys who were in the TAP group with him. The girls in the group began to look out for him. In his end-of-TAP-project review, James stated, "It was the best thing I have ever done forever. I would recommend that other people do it, too, but only if they take me with them!"

Playfulness arises out of the nonverbal give and take, the action and reaction during these sessions. This leads to interaction and the beginnings of relationship building, the precursor to developing and sustaining positive attachments. As Almon (2013) has stated, "Play-deprived children fail to know themselves and the world around them with the depth available to the playful child. Play also serves the important purpose of showing [them] . . . life can be fun even though it is often rich with difficulties" (p. 6).

Others have spoken about the role of body and physical connection in relationships. "Children's need for contact and connection with others is deep-seated and utilizes our innate musicality based on early rhythm and movement so that we exist not as a body alone, but form relationships through and with our body or as our body" (Chown, 2014).

As children explore their innate physicality, they can be both noisy and busy, inquiring and speculative, free ranging and focused. All of these were operating with James in his experience with the horses and his peers. As Tovey (2007) notes, "Laughter, gleefulness, whooping and shrieking with delight are characteristics of young children's play, and contribute to a sense of outdoors as a place of joy where children can be literally and metaphorically 'giddy with glee' " (p. 21). Being outdoors with the horses during the TAP program provided James with this powerful experience within himself while connecting with the horses and the other humans who were there.

Case 2: Myra

Myra was 6 years old and in first grade. Both of her parents had been killed in a car accident 6 months prior to her coming for therapy. She had lived with her grandmother, with whom she spoke, but she refused to speak with anyone else outside the home. The school was concerned that her selective mutism was interfering with her social development and her ability to learn. She had seen another play therapist who had used both child-centered play therapy as well as some more directive activities with her, and she had mostly remained seated in a corner with her back turned to the therapist. The therapist noted that she sometimes looked around at the toys with interest, but she seemed unable to explore the playroom, even when the therapist invited her to do so. She cooperated with the directive activities minimally. When asked to draw, she did so, but she covered her paper and again turned her back. The therapist, when referring her to me (RV) for AAPT said that their sessions had been painful because Myra was so closed off. The therapist had tried to create a safe and accepting atmosphere, but after eight sessions, nothing had changed. While FT can be helpful in cases such as this, the grandmother had some serious medical issues that precluded that from happening at this time.

Myra did not talk with me during her first sessions. I started by talking about how to meet dogs safely, and then demonstrated that approach with a life-size stuffed toy dog. I asked Myra to do the same thing I had done, and I animated the toy dog in a playful manner. She smiled shyly, and did as I had done, but said nothing. There was no pressure put on her to talk at all. I then shared a letter that my primary AAPT dog, Kirrie, had "written" to her to explain that Kirrie liked to play with children, and then we met Kirrie in person. Myra used what we had just practiced, and I saw that she was trying not to smile. Kirrie's wagging tail swung her entire back end, and I commented, "Wow! Kirrie is really excited to meet you! Do you see how her back end is wiggling?" Myra looked at me quickly, then looked away, but again there was a smile. Kirrie licked her cheek, and again Myra smiled. I then showed Myra how to do the "kiss me" cue, where Kirrie would touch her nose to Myra's hand. It's a way to redirect Kirrie's licking behavior, as many children have mixed feelings about licks—they like the attention from the dog, but not necessarily the messiness of the licks.

Kirrie, like most dogs, learns gestural cues rapidly. An outstretched flat hand is her cue to touch her nose to the palm. She also knows verbal cues for each of her trained behaviors, so saying "Kiss me" also brings the response. In Myra's case, I said, "Kirrie knows lots of things to do, and you can show her a sign about what you want her to do, or you can tell her what you want. It's totally up to you which way you do it!" Myra was now much more engaged with the process and with me, so I taught her four simple behaviors, using both the gestures and the words as I did so. Then, I told her that she could try whichever of these that she wanted. She used only the gestural cues and Kirrie played along with her usual enthusiasm. For most of the rest of the session, I stood back and simply reflected what was happening and how Myra seemed to feel: "You're having Kirrie do another 'down' and 'stay.' Kirrie is trying to do what you've asked. That's fun to see Kirrie do what you tell her." At times, I empathically responded through Kirrie: "Kirrie, Myra is really showing you what she wants you to do. Myra is having a good time with you!" By the end of the first session, Myra was absorbed in her interactions with Kirrie and had visibly relaxed her posture. When I told her it was time to leave but that she could come back if she wished, she looked at me squarely and nodded her head yes.

The second session was similar to the first, as Myra remembered all of the cues I had shown her, and she asked Kirrie to do them all for her again. I remained relatively nondirective throughout, reflecting the actions and feelings being expressed. Myra also looked around the room and showed Kirrie some of the toys. Again, I used empathic listening during this play: "You're showing Kirrie some of the toys. Kirrie, Myra wants you to see the different things in here. Myra is thinking about playing with some of them." The latter sentence reflected what I was seeing in Myra's nonverbal behaviors. Myra then did play briefly with some of the toys, mostly looking to see how they worked, showing them to Kirrie, and then putting them back where they had been. I continued using mostly nondirective skills throughout. Myra did not speak during this session either, but I could see her relaxing and exploring the playroom and her budding relationship with Kirrie more fully.

In the third session, I started with a more directive intervention. I showed her how to use a clicker and treats to communicate with Kirrie, and I asked if she wanted to help Kirrie learn a new trick. She nodded enthusiastically. Because she had relaxed considerably during the prior session, I thought that adding a somewhat more directive activity that involved communication and further engagement with the dog might be useful. I gave Myra three choices of simple tricks we could train, and although she still was not verbal, I knew I had her full attention. She nodded eagerly, pointed to things she wanted me to see, and was fully engaged nonverbally. My goal was not to get her to speak, but to connect with her, and this was happening.

Myra and I then used some simple clicker training to teach Kirrie to touch a sticky note with her paw. Kirrie had never done this before, but she had learned paw targeting with a closet light and with cloth napkins, so the concept was familiar to her. We started with a large piece of paper, and Myra clicked and gave a treat every time Kirrie's front paw touched the paper. After cutting the paper in half for a few trials, we were able to have Kirrie touch the sticky note on the floor. We then added some sticky notes and taught Kirrie to touch several of them, one at a time.

At that point, I said that it was time to give a name to this game. I asked Myra if she had any ideas for a name, and she shook her head no. She was not yet ready to speak. I moved right on, saying, "Well, I bet you've heard of the game Mother May I? haven't you?" She nodded. "I think we should call this game Myra Says Touch the Note!—is that a good name?" She nodded yes, with a big smile. I demonstrated, saying "Myra says touch the note" before giving Kirrie the gestural cue, and Myra continued to click and treat. I told Myra that now Kirrie needed her help to practice this. I matter-of-factly said, "How you help her is up to you. You can show her with your hand, or you can say 'Myra says touch the note!' or you can do both—it's totally up to you! You are doing just great with the clicker and giving her those treats, and look how eager she is to try this with you!" Again, the focus was on removing all pressure to use words while opening the opportunity to do so if she chose.

The first several times, Myra continued with the gestural cues, the clicks, and treats. Then I heard her whisper, "Myra says touch the note!" to Kirrie. I continued to reflect on what was happening and provided encouragement and praise as I had been (this was still considered a directive AAPT session even though I was using many nondirective skills), such as "You're practicing with Kirrie. Kirrie's really paying attention to you. Nice job with that clicker!" and then, in a quiet reflection, "You just told Kirrie the name of the game, and now she is wanting to play it again and again with you! You're really helping her learn." For the remainder of that session, Myra used quiet words to give the verbal cue before the gestural cue, and her voice became louder and stronger by the end of the session. Kirrie kept her focus entirely on Myra, and Myra went to her grandmother in the waiting area at the end and said, "Myra says touch the note!" Rather than meeting for a quick update with the grandmother at the end, I decided the best use of that time was to do a quick demonstration with the grandmother. We all went back into the playroom, and Myra demonstrated what Kirrie had learned. Even though she spoke with the grandmother at home, when we did the demonstration, she began with just gestural cues again, but after three trials, we both heard her whisper the name of the game to the dog. She continued to whisper it in a low voice for the rest of the demonstration. The grandmother was very pleased, telling me privately that this was the first time since the accident that anyone other than she had heard Myra speak.

From the next session on, Myra began speaking to Kirrie in a normal tone of voice, and our sessions continued without incident. Myra loved teaching Kirrie new things, demonstrating them for her grandmother, and making videos of them. I had been in touch with the school from the start, asking that her teachers and counselor refrain from any efforts to get her to talk, and providing some guidance on how to handle various situations. After Myra's fifth session of AAPT, she began whispering to her teacher, and within a matter of weeks began speaking regularly at school with her teachers and classmates.

Myra continued in AAPT as she dealt with the loss of her parents. She and Kirrie created a book that contained stories and photos and drawings in memory of her parents. Kirrie watched as she created some sandtrays about her parents and their accident. A modified version of FT was used to accommodate her grandmother's medical needs, and that helped their own relationship grow in positive ways while Myra continued to work out the many feelings she had been holding inside. She continued to do well at home and at school. At the end of therapy, she painted a picture of Kirrie on a special thank-you card . She asked me to help her write the words on it: "Kirrie, thank you for talking with me. You are a great trick dog. Remember the tricks I taught you."

Case 3: David

David was an 11-year-old boy who had significant vision problems; because of this, he had impaired ability to read other people's facial expressions and body language. As a result, he was quiet and with-drawn. He came to the TAP program with a group of other children. As with James (Case 1), he did not speak but seemed to enjoy the sessions. He had not spoken by the third session, but he spent considerable time grooming the horses and touching them. He eagerly picked up the brushes and worked hard for a long time brushing them.

In the third session, I (TF-T) used an EAGALA (Equine Assisted Growth and Learning Association; *www.eagala.org*) activity called Extended Appendages. Here, teams of three children link their arms together. The person in the middle is "the brain," and only the brain can speak; the two on either side are "the appendages." They can move only under the direction of the brain, and the brain must specify the left arm and leg and the right arm and leg to complete certain tasks. The activity is to stay in this configuration and to catch a horse, put a halter on its head, groom it, put on a saddle and fasten it. The children got into their teams, and David was selected to be the brain in the middle of one of them. My cofacilitator and I wondered how this was going to work, but as one does in play therapy, decided simply to trust the process.

As soon as the teams linked arms, only the brains could speak. Immediately, Buster, one of the Arabian horses, came right over to David's team and tried to kiss David. (The horses have been trained to kiss by taking carrots out of people's mouths very gently, and even though David didn't have a carrot, Buster chose this time to check it out!) David was surprised and was unable to push Buster away because his arms were linked. He smiled, laughed, and very quietly but clearly told his left arm what to do to prevent Buster from kissing any more. From there on, he directed his team extremely well as they worked on the task, and when things went wrong, he laughed aloud. The horses kept returning to nudge the brains of the teams, accompanied by much laughter and screams of delight from the children. David's team, under his verbal direction, achieved their goal first among all the teams. They were delighted and spontaneously hugged Buster and then each other. From there, David remained soft-spoken but much more verbal and interactive. His school and parents reported that he was much more confident and assertive in school thereafter.

Case 4: Lara

Lara was 16 years old and angry. Her parents had divorced when she was 13, and it had not been amicable. She had been placed in the middle of them, asked to choose between them, and had been subjected to both of them badmouthing the other to her. She had been devastated by their breakup, and the nastiness that ensued had turned her pain into anger. More recently, her father had moved across the country, and she visited him each summer. The move had decreased the open animosity between them, but she was still aware of simmering tensions.

Lara had been a handful for her mother, who was worried about her rebelliousness becoming more extreme. Her mother was seeing another therapist and she and Lara's father had attended some coparenting sessions just before he moved. These had seemed to help them get along better, at least in Lara's presence.

Lara made it clear that she didn't want to talk about her family. She described it as "a mess." She expressed interest in animals and agreed to AAPT sessions with me (RV). I used a variety of AAPT interventions with her, all of which seemed to work well. Even so, she did not share much of herself during the sessions, and seemed to avoid any conversations where she might have to share her feelings. When I reflected her feelings during the sessions, she often gave me a sharp look and then denied that she felt that way. Although my reflections seemed quite accurate, they felt threatening to her, so I cut back on them and underplayed the feeling vocabulary in an effort to retain the safety of the sessions for her. Below, I discuss an activity that seemed to allow her to let go of some of her anger and begin dealing with the pain beneath.

In our fifth AAPT session, I told her we could help Kirrie with her "balancing act." This was a spur-of-the-moment idea I had when Lara briefly said her parents had been acting up again. She didn't want to give details because she just wanted to be with Kirrie. I did not push.

Kirrie has always been a very athletic dog, so I thought this might be possible for her to do. Lara had taken gymnastic lessons until the last year, and I told her that Kirrie needed to learn the "balance beam." I mentioned how much Kirrie liked learning new things and that this might help her stay in shape. The storyline developed as I handed Lara a stack of printer paper (8 ½ x 11 inches), and asked her to create a path on the playroom floor. After she did so, I told her that this was a path through some craggy, rough mountains, and she and Kirrie had to stay on the road without "falling off" to reach the other side of the treacherous mountain pass. She could use treats and one other prop—anything she chose in the room. The main thing was that she had to walk on the paper and help Kirrie walk behind her. I defined "falling off" the path as when both of her feet or all four of Kirrie's feet were off the paper trail. She laughed and asked me what would happen if one of them fell off. I playfully shrugged and asked, "What do you think?" She said they would have to start over, and I said that made sense to me. To add a little more to the lightness of the session, I said that the starting point was the hospital, and the end point was a safe, fun, friendly place where they could relax and do things they really liked to do.

At first, Lara had trouble keeping on the paper trail, and sometimes Kirrie would wander off to another part of the room. I stood back and smiled, just observing as she did some problem solving. When they "fell off" I groaned and said things like, "Oh noooooo! They're back in the hospital again!! I wonder how many broken bones they have THIS time?!?!" Lara thought this was very funny.

On their fourth attempt, Lara loaded her pockets with dog treats, and she began feeding them to Kirrie every two or three steps. She placed them behind her knee when feeding Kirrie to keep Kirrie directly behind her. In a couple places, she began to lose her balance, laughing. I commented, "It's so hard to keep your balance between these two steep cliffs!" At first she said it was impossible, then added, "Well, maybe not IMPOSSIBLE." I added, "It's pretty tough when every move could be a false move, though." She nodded and continued on her journey.

She completed the trip across the mountain pass and landed in the safe and fun place. I put on a tangled blonde wig and picked up a magic wand. In a mock-princess voice I said, "Welcome to the land of choices! You and your lovely dog get to make one wish each, and if my wand isn't too rusty, perhaps I can grant your wish." By this time, she was fully engaged in this imaginary dramatic play therapy scenario. She thought for a minute and said, "Kirrie wants to play b-a-l-l." (She had already learned that Kirrie got very excited if she heard the word *ball*.) She then said, "As for me, I just wish I could have some fun with my mom without her worrying about my dad." I reflected these wishes, still retaining the magical princess persona. The princess said, "Ahhhh. What a clever wish! Perhaps you can speak with that other woman who was here a minute ago [referring to my "real" self] to see if she has any ideas for that!"

As we stopped the activity, got out Kirrie's ball, and shared a laugh, we spoke of how good she felt solving that puzzle. I said that perhaps we could demonstrate for her mother the following week. Lara brightened and said, "I have a better idea! We can have my mother do it, too!" A plan was hatched!

We involved her mother the following week, and Lara and she had some fun together. This opened the door for me to do some family AAPT with both of them. Kirrie was not always involved in our sessions, but I often suggested tasks for the two of them to do together, each with a bit of a challenge included. We also spent a little time talking about their relationship during part of these sessions, and we incorporated some other family play therapy activities. Soon, they planned at least one fun activity each week to share at home or in the community.

As Lara and her mother rebuilt their relationship with more playfulness and enjoyable times together, the need for therapy stopped. They both had enjoyed the dog so much that they decided that they would become dog walkers for the local humane organization. They were not yet ready for a dog of their own, but they had found common interests to pursue. Lara's mother's confidence grew as their relationship grew, and she felt less threatened by her ex-husband's relationship with Lara. Things began moving in a better direction. In this case, Lara's ability to connect safely with Kirrie allowed her to accept more playfulness in her sessions. This, in turn, allowed her to find ways to drop some of her anger and express her longing for a better relationship with her mother. This also was made more possible through AAPT family sessions. Lara never had to talk about her angry feelings to get past them. She needed to be empowered to take some action to change things for herself. AAPT allowed that to happen through the playful activities and challenges with Kirrie.

CONCLUSION

AAPT represents a true integration of play therapy with AAT, harnessing the power of play along with that of appropriately selected and trained animals. Both forms of therapy create a sense of emotional safety that frees clients to be themselves and to feel good about themselves, and the combination seems to hasten the trust and empowerment that clients develop. The animals bring their unique selves to the process, and the therapist processes the special moments that the clients have with the animals using the many tools of play therapy and effective therapy skills. Clients need not process their struggles verbally, but they often play out in their interactions with the animals.

The emergent field of AAPT requires substantial training and supervised practice to ensure its effectiveness in achieving desired therapy outcomes while preserving the well-being of the animals. Since many animals enjoy play as much as children do, AAPT provides a safe opportunity for all participants to develop relationships, express needs, use empathy, and solve problems. Animals often seem safer than humans, especially when children are hurt or upset with the people in their lives. Play creates an opportunity for relaxation, bonding, exploration, and resolution. Although much more research is needed, clinical outcomes and preliminary studies have consistently shown that clients show behavioral improvements within a few sessions, and clients and their families or teachers report noticeable positive changes in a short time as well. It seems well worth it to invest the time and learning required to be an ethically sound practitioner.

Children who clam up typically are anxious. They want someone to understand them, but they fear the consequences if they let their needs be known. Some are unsure of an unfamiliar therapy experience. Others struggle with the loss of control in their lives. Sometimes they are trying to cope with the damage caused by abuse and attachment disruptions. Some simply are shy or lack social competence. Whatever their reasons, reticent children seem to do well when animals are brought into the picture. They relate to the animals readily, and they begin to relax. They learn to trust the therapist, almost by proxy.

For therapists interested in learning more about AAPT, the International Institute for AAPT (*www.iiaapt.org*) offers training, supervision, and a mental health certification in this exciting field.

FIVE RECOMMENDED PRACTICES

1. Obtain training and competence in animal behavior/ethology, play therapy, and AAPT and apply current knowledge of animal science to select, socialize, train, and engage animals appropriate to the work. Determine the form and level of structure of AAPT that best meet the child's needs and goals.

2. Allow and encourage client exploration/seeking with the animal to use the seeking system of the brain for healing and maintain a light and playful atmosphere to ensure emotional safety.

3. Observe animal body language with fluency in real time to ensure animal welfare and modeling of humane treatment.

4. Incorporate the social lubrication effects of animals to engage the child and harness and acknowledge his or her strengths when interacting with the animal. Guide the child to build a mutually respectful and healthy attachment relationship with the animal and ensure goodness of fit for the child and for the animal.

5. Incorporate touch and free, nondirected play to harness the oxytocin effects of human–animal interactions. Give child choices to interact verbally or nonverbally with the animal for empowerment.

REFERENCES

Almon, J. (2013). *Adventure: The value of risk in children's play*. Annapolis, MD: Alliance for Childhood.

Chandler, C. K. (2012). *Animal assisted therapy in counseling* (2nd ed.). New York: Routledge.

Chown, A. (2014). *Play therapy in the outdoors: Taking play therapy out of the playroom and into natural environments*. London: Jessica Kingsley.

Fine, A. H. (Ed.). (2015). *Handbook on animal-assisted therapy: Foundations and guidelines for animal-assisted interventions* (4th ed.). London: Academic Press/Elsevier.

Jalongo, M. R. (Ed.). (2014). *Teaching compassion: Humane education in early childhood*. New York: Springer.

Louv, R. (2008). *Last child in the woods: Saving our children from nature-deficit disorder*. Chapel Hill, NC: Algonquin Books.

Malchiodi, C. A. (Ed.). (2015). *Creative interventions with traumatized children* (2nd ed.). New York: Guilford Press.

Melson, G. F. (2001). *Why the wild things are: Animals in the lives of children*. Cambridge, MA: Harvard University Press.

Melson, G. F., & Fine, A. H. (2015). Animals in the lives of children. In A. H. Fine (Ed.), *Handbook on animal-assisted therapy: Foundations and guidelines for animal-assisted interventions* (4th ed., pp. 179–194). London: Academic Press/Elsevier.

Morell, V. (2014). "Love hormone" has same effect on humans and dogs. Retrieved June 9, 2014, from *news.sciencemag.org/brain-behavior/2014;06/love-hormone-has-same-effect-humans-and-dogs*.

Olmert, M. D. (2009). *Made for each other: The biology of the human-animal bond*. Cambridge, MA: Da Capo Press.

Olmert, M. D. (2010). "Dog good." The latest on the biology of the human–animal bond. Retrieved May 5, 2010, from *www.psychologytoday.com/blog/made-each-other/201005/dog-good*.

Parish-Plass, N. (Ed.). (2013). *Animal-assisted psychotherapy: Theory, issues, and practice*. West Lafayette, IN: Purdue University Press.

Sheppard, C. H. (1998). *Brave Bart: A story for traumatized and grieving children*. Grosse Pointe Woods, MI: Institute for Trauma and Loss in Children.

Tovey, H. (2007). *Playing outdoors: Spaces and places, risks and challenges*. Berkshire, UK: Open University Press.

Trotter, K. S. (2012). *Harnessing the power of equine assisted counseling: Adding animal assisted therapy to your practice*. New York: Routledge.

VanFleet, R. (2008). *Play therapy with kids & canines: Benefits for children's developmental and psychosocial health*. Sarasota, FL: Professional Resource Press.

VanFleet, R. (2015a). *Animal Assisted Play Therapy: Theory, research, and practice* (4th ed.) [Training manual]. Boiling Springs, PA: Play Therapy Press.

VanFleet, R. (2015b). *The creative play therapy process* (4th ed.) [Training manual]. Boiling Springs, PA: Play Therapy Press.

VanFleet, R., & Faa-Thompson, T. (2010). The case for using Animal Assisted Play Therapy. *British Journal of Play Therapy, 6,* 4–18.

VanFleet, R., & Faa-Thompson, T. (2014). Including animals in play therapy with young children and families. In M. R. Jalongo (Ed.), *Teaching compassion: Humane education in early childhood* (pp. 89–107). New York: Springer.

VanFleet, R., & Faa-Thompson, T. (2015a). Animal-assisted play therapy. In D. A. Crenshaw & A. L. Stewart (Eds.), *Play therapy: A comprehensive guide to theory and practice* (pp. 201–214). New York: Guilford Press.

VanFleet, R., & Faa-Thompson, T. (2015b). Animal-assisted play therapy to empower vulnerable children. In E. J. Green & A. C. Myrick (Eds.), *Play therapy with vulnerable populations: No child forgotten* (pp. 85–103). Lanham, MD: Rowman & Littlefield.

VanFleet, R., & Faa-Thompson, T. (2015c). Short-term animal-assisted play therapy for children. In H. G. Kaduson & C. E. Schaefer (Eds.), *Short-term play therapy for children* (3rd ed., pp. 175–197). New York: Guilford Press.

VanFleet, R., & Faa-Thompson, T. (2017). *Animal assisted play therapy.* Sarasota, FL: Professional Resource Press.

VanFleet, R., Fine, A. H., O'Callaghan, D., Mackintosh, T., & Gimeno, J. (2015). Application of animal-assisted interventions in professional settings: An overview of alternatives. In A. H. Fine (Ed.), *Handbook on animal-assisted therapy: Foundations and guidelines for animal-assisted interventions* (4th ed., pp. 157–177). London: Academic Press/Elsevier.

VanFleet, R., Sywulak, A. E., & Sniscak, C. C. (2010). *Child-centered play therapy.* New York: Guilford Press.

Zak, P. (2014). Dogs (and cats) can love. Retrieved April 22, 2014, from *www.theatlantic.com/health/archive/2014/04/does-your-dog-or-cat-actually-love-you/360784/access.*

Index

Note: *f*, *t*, or *n* following a page number indicates a figure, table, or note.